SPRINGHOUSE NOTES

Critical Care and Emergency Nursing

Third Edition

Sandra Smith Huddleston, RN, PhD, CCRN
Assistant Professor of Nursing
Berea College
Berea, Kentucky

Sondra G. Ferguson, RN, MSN, CS, CCRN
Clinical Nurse Specialist for Critical Care
Department of Veterans Affairs, VA Medical Center
Lexington, Kentucky

Springhouse Corporation
Springhouse, Pennsylvania

Staff

Executive Director
Matthew Cahill

Editorial Director
June Norris

Art Director
John Hubbard

Managing Editor
David Moreau

Acquisitions Editors
Patricia Kardish Fischer, RN, BSN; Louise Quinn

Clinical Consultant
Maryann Foley, RN, BSN

Editors
Naina Chohan, Karen Diamond, Michael Shaw

Copy Editors
Cynthia C. Breuninger (manager), Christine Cunniffe, Stacey A. Follin, Brenna Mayer, Pamela Wingrod

Designers
Arlene Putterman (associate art director), Lesley Weissman-Cook (book designer), Joseph Clark, Elaine Ezrow, Jacalyn Facciolo, Donald G. Knauss

Production Coordinator
Margaret A. Rastiello

Editorial Assistants
Beverly Lane, Mary Madden, Jeanne Napier

Manufacturing
Deborah Meiris (director), Pat Dorshaw (manager), T.A. Landis

---

The clinical procedures described and recommended in this publication are based on research and consultation with nursing, medical, and legal authorities. To the best of our knowledge, these procedures reflect currently accepted practice; nevertheless, they can't be considered absolute and universal recommendations. For individual application, all recommendations must be considered in light of the patient's clinical condition and, before administration of new or infrequently used drugs, in light of the latest package-insert information. The author and the publisher disclaim responsibility for any adverse effects resulting directly or indirectly from any suggested procedures herein, from any undetected errors, or from the reader's misunderstanding of the text.

Printed in the United States of America.

SNCE3-020897

A member of the Reed Elsevier plc group

Library of Congress Cataloging-in-Publication Data
Huddleston, Sandra Smith.
Critical care and emergency nursing / Sandra Smith Huddleston, Sondra G. Ferguson. — 3rd ed.
p. cm. — (Springhouse notes)
Includes bibliographical references and index.
1. Intensive care nursing. 2. Emergency nursing. I. Ferguson,Sondra G. II. Title. III. Series
[DNLM: 1. Critical Illness—nursing—outlines. 2. Emergencies—nursing—outlines. 3. Critical Care—outlines. 4. Emergency Nursing—outlines. WY 18.2 H884c 1997] RT120.I5H83 1997
610.73'61—dc21
DNLM/DLC for Library of Congress 96-40890
ISBN 0-87434-900-1 (alk. paper) CIP

Contents

Appendices

Advisory Board and Reviewers

ADVISORY BOARD

Mildred Wernet Boyd, RN, MSN, MSA
Associate Professor of Nursing
Essex Community College
Baltimore

Dorothy Brooten, PhD, FAAN
Associate Dean of Research and Graduate Studies
Frances Payne Bolton School of Nursing
Case Western Reserve University
Cleveland

Lillian S. Brunner, RN, MSN, ScD, FAAN
Nurse-Author
Brunner Associates, Inc.
Lancaster, Pa.

Irma J. D'Antonio, RN, PhD
Chairperson, Department of Family Nursing
University of North Carolina at Charlotte

Kathleen Dracup, RN, DNSc, FAAN
Professor and Hassenplug Chair of Nursing
University of California at Los Angeles

Cecile A. Lengacher, RN, PhD
Associate Professor
College of Nursing
University of South Florida
Tampa

Barbara L. Tower, RN, MA, MSN, CCRN
Professor of Nursing
Essex Community College
Baltimore

REVIEWERS

Linda S. Baas, RN, PhD, CCRN
Assistant Professor
College of Nursing and Health
University of Cincinnati
Cincinnati

Carrie A. McCoy, RN, MSN, CEN
Associate Professor of Nursing
Northern Kentucky University
Highland Heights

Leanna R. Miller, RN, MN, CCRN, CEN, CPNP
Pediatric Nurse Practitioner
Clinical Nurse Specialist
Medical Center of Central Georgia
Macon

Michaelene P. Mirr, RN, PhD, CCRN
Associate Professor of Nursing
University of Wisconsin
Eau Claire

How to Use Springhouse Notes

Springhouse Notes is a multi-volume study guide series developed especially for nursing students. Each volume provides essential course material in an outline format, enabling the student to review information efficiently.

Special features appear in every chapter to make information accessible and easy to remember. **Learning objectives** encourage the student to evaluate knowledge before and after study. **Chapter overview** highlights the chapter's major concepts. Within the outlined text, key points appear in color to facilitate a quick review of critical information. Key points may include cardinal signs and symptoms, current theories, important steps in a nursing procedure, critical assessment findings, crucial nursing interventions, or successful therapies and treatments. **Points to remember** summarize each chapter's major themes. **Study questions** then offer another opportunity to review material and assess knowledge gained before moving on to new information. **Critical thinking and application exercises** conclude each chapter, challenging students to expand on knowledge gained.

Other features appear throughout the book to facilitate learning: **Teaching tips** highlight key areas to address with patient teaching. **Clinical alerts** point out essential information on how to provide safe, effective care. **Decision trees** promote critical thinking. Difficult, frequently used, or sometimes misunderstood terms are indicated by SMALL CAPITAL LETTERS in the outline and defined in the glossary, Appendix A; answers to the study questions appear in Appendix B. Finally, a brand-new Windows-based software program (see diskette on inside back cover) poses 100 multiple-choice questions in random or sequential order to assess your knowledge.

The Springhouse Notes volumes are designed as learning tools, not as primary information sources. When read conscientiously as a supplement to class attendance and textbook reading, Springhouse Notes can enhance understanding and help improve test scores and final grades.

CHAPTER

1

Perspectives on Critical Care and Emergency Nursing

Learning objectives

After studying this chapter, you should be able to:

- Identify general principles related to patients requiring critical care and emergency nursing.
- Differentiate among the independent, dependent, and interdependent interventions of critical care and emergency nurses.
- Describe the concept of triage in emergency nursing.
- Discuss the roles and functions of critical care and emergency nurses.
- Name legal and ethical issues that can affect critical care or emergency nursing.

Chapter overview

Critical care and emergency nurses are specialists who possess greater knowledge and skills than nurse generalists. The practice of critical care and emergency nursing requires priority and triage decision making, often in life-threatening and unpredictable situations. Ethical and legal issues impact the independent, dependent, and interdependent interventions of the critical care and emergency nurse.

♦ I. Introduction

A. Scope of practice
   1. Critical care nursing and emergency nursing are separate specialties with the common goal of restoring physiologic or psychological stability to the severely ill patient
   2. Because these two nursing specialties encompass all areas of practice, critical care and emergency nurses must have knowledge and skill beyond those of the nurse generalist
      a. Both have a core knowledge of principles and techniques that apply to medicine, surgery, pediatrics, obstetrics, and psychiatry
      b. Both have core concepts that are essential components of adequate assessment and appropriate therapy
      c. Both use the nursing process as a framework for practice

B. Nursing interventions
   1. Critical care nursing and emergency nursing encompass independent, dependent, and interdependent interventions
      a. *Independent* nursing interventions are unique to nursing and include management of the environment, teaching, counseling, and initiating referrals
      b. *Dependent* nursing interventions are prescribed by appropriate health care personnel
      c. *Interdependent* nursing interventions are determined by multidisciplinary collaboration
   2. Critical care and emergency nurses are often responsible for making life-and-death decisions, placing them at a high legal risk
      a. Priorities must be determined quickly, based on sound knowledge and judgment
      b. TRIAGE decisions must be made to expedite care
   3. Critical care and emergency nurses are at high risk of injury from possible exposure to infections, such as hepatitis, acquired immunodeficiency syndrome, and other communicable diseases

♦ II. Critical care nursing

A. General information
   1. Critical care nursing deals with human responses to life-threatening problems and includes the critically ill patient, the critical care nurse, and the critical care environment
   2. Care is provided to patients of all ages with alterations in physical or emotional health
   3. The critically ill patient is at high risk for developing life-threatening problems and requires constant, intensive, multidisciplinary assessment and intervention to restore stability, prevent complications, and achieve and maintain optimal responses

4. The critical care nurse coordinates interventions aimed at resolving life-threatening problems

B. Historical development
   1. Critical care began as a component of recovery rooms before expanding into coronary care units in the 1960s
   2. The American Association of Critical-Care Nurses (AACN) was organized in 1969
   3. A competency-based examination was developed in 1975 to provide certification in critical care nursing; certification is valid for 3 years; available for adult, neonatal, and pediatric certification
   4. The AACN developed Standards for Nursing Care of the Critically Ill in 1981 to explain the role of the critical care nurse in ensuring quality care for critically ill patients and their families

C. Critical care environment
   1. Units may be specifically designated as medical, surgical, coronary, pediatric, neonatal, recovery, or postanesthesia or may encompass other areas in some institutions
   2. Adequate resources (emergency equipment, supplies, and support systems) are necessary for safe care
   3. A management and administrative structure is required to ensure effective care through all phases of the patient's hospital stay, from emergency department (ED) to discharge
   4. Legal, regulatory, social, economic, and political trends must be monitored to promote the early recognition of problems and a timely response
   5. Specialized electronic technology and techniques are used to monitor patient status continuously; these may create safety hazards for patients, such as possible exposure to electric shock

D. Roles of the critical care nurse
   1. Care provider: provides comprehensive — and at times highly technical — direct care to the patient and family in response to life-threatening health problems
   2. Educator: provides the patient and family with education based on their learning needs and ability and on the severity of the situation; allows the patient to assume more responsibility for meeting health care needs as his condition stabilizes or improves
   3. Manager: coordinates the care provided by various health care workers to provide optimal nursing care to critically ill patients
   4. Advocate: protects the patient's rights

E. Functions of the critical care nurse
   1. Assesses and implements treatment for patient responses to life-threatening health problems
   2. Provides direct measures to resuscitate, if necessary

3. Uses independent, dependent, and interdependent interventions to restore stability, prevent complications, and achieve and maintain optimal patient responses
4. Provides health education to the patient and family
5. Supervises patient care and ancillary personnel
6. Supports patient adaptation, restores health, and preserves the patient's rights, including the right to refuse treatment

F. Legal issues affecting the provision of critical care nursing
1. Negligence
2. MALPRACTICE
3. INFORMED CONSENT
4. Implied consent
5. Advanced directives, including DURABLE POWER OF ATTORNEY and living wills

G. Ethical issues affecting the provision of critical care nursing
1. Ethnic and religious doctrines that limit treatment options
2. Allocation of resources that may limit admissions or promote premature discharges
3. Use of critical care beds for terminally ill patients
4. Discontinuation of resuscitation or life-support measures
5. Do-not-resuscitate (DNR) orders

♦ III. Emergency nursing

A. General information
1. Emergency nursing addresses human responses to any trauma or sudden illness that requires interventions ranging from minimal care to life support
2. Care is provided in any setting to people of all ages with actual or perceived alterations in physical or emotional health
3. Initially, patients may not have a medical diagnosis
4. Care is *episodic* when patients return frequently, *primary* when it is the initial option for health or preventive care, and *acute* when patients need immediate and additional interventions

B. Historical development
1. Florence Nightingale was the first emergency nurse, providing care to the wounded in the Crimean War in 1854
2. The Emergency Department Nurses Association (EDNA) was organized in 1970
3. A competency-based examination, first administered in 1980, provides Certification in Emergency Nursing for 4 years
4. EDNA developed Standards of Emergency Nursing Practice, published in 1983, to be used as a guideline for excellence and outcome criteria against which performance is measured and evaluated

5. EDNA changed its name to the Emergency Nurses Association in 1985 to encompass a practice setting larger than the ED

C. Emergency care environment
1. Prehospital care by emergency medical services (EMS), emergency medical technicians, and paramedics provides initial stabilization and transport of patients; flight nurses provide care during prehospital and intrahospital transport; personnel communicate with the ED during patient transport
2. The national emergency telephone number 911 is the result of an effort to improve access to EMS
3. The concept of the emergency room has expanded to that of the ED, which provides various levels of care
4. Specialized electronic technology and techniques are used to monitor patient status continuously; they may pose safety hazards to patients, such as possible exposure to electric shock

D. Triage
1. Triage classifies patients for assessment and treatment priorities
2. Triage decisions require the rapid and effective gathering of objective and subjective data to determine the type of priority situation
3. *Emergent situations* are potentially life-threatening; they include such conditions as respiratory distress or arrest, cardiac arrest, severe chest pain, seizures, hemorrhage, severe trauma resulting in open chest or abdominal wounds, shock, poisonings, drug overdoses, temperatures over 105° F (40.5° C), emergency childbirth, and delivery complications
4. *Urgent situations* are serious but not life-threatening if treatment is delayed briefly
   a. They include such conditions as chest pain without respiratory distress, major fractures, burns, decreased level of consciousness, back injuries, nausea or vomiting, severe abdominal pain, temperature between 102° and 105° F (38.9° and 40.5° C), bleeding from any orifice, acute panic, and anxiety

CLINICAL ALERT

   b. The severity of temperature elevation is related to age; the young often have temperature elevations in the moderate range without other symptoms, whereas elderly people may not have a temperature elevation greater than 101° F and be extremely ill
5. *Nonemergency situations* are not acute and are considered minor to moderately severe; they include chronic backache or other symptoms, moderate headache, minor burns, fractures, sprains, and upper respiratory tract or urinary infections

E. Roles of the emergency nurse
1. Care provider: provides comprehensive direct care to the patient and family

2. Educator: provides patient and family with education based on their learning needs and ability and on the severity of the situation and allows the patient to assume more responsibility for meeting health care needs
3. Manager: coordinates activities of others in the multidisciplinary team to achieve the specific goal of providing emergency care
4. Advocate: ensures protection of the patient's rights

F. Functions of the emergency nurse
1. Uses triage to determine priorities based on assessment and anticipation of the patient's needs
2. Provides direct measures to resuscitate, if necessary
3. Provides preliminary care before the patient is transferred to the primary care area
4. Provides health education to the patient and family
5. Supervises patient care and ancillary personnel
6. Provides support and protection for the patient and family

G. Legal issues affecting the provision of emergency nursing
1. Negligence
2. Malpractice
3. Good Samaritan laws (these statutes may protect private citizens but usually do not apply to emergency personnel on duty or in normal emergency situations)
4. Informed consent
5. Implied consent
6. Duty to report suspected crimes to the police
7. Duty to gather evidence in criminal investigations; be aware of hospital policy and state laws for evidence collection
8. Advanced directives, including durable power of attorney and living wills

H. Ethical issues affecting the provision of emergency nursing
1. Ethnic and religious doctrines that limit treatment options
2. Allocation of emergency care resources that may limit admissions or promote premature discharges
3. Decisions to stop resuscitation efforts or to resuscitate terminal cases
4. Living wills

POINTS TO REMEMBER

- Critical care nursing and emergency nursing have a common goal of restoring physiologic or psychological stability to a critically ill patient.

- Triage decisions require the rapid and effective gathering of objective and subjective data.
- Critical care nursing and emergency nursing are high-risk occupations from a legal standpoint.
- Ethical dilemmas affect the provision of care for critically ill and emergency patients.

STUDY QUESTIONS

To evaluate your understanding of this chapter, answer the following questions in the space provided; then compare your responses with the correct answers in Appendix B, page 279.

1. Which factors help make critical care and emergency nursing high-risk areas of practice? ______________________________

   ____

   ____

2. Which three areas of critical care nursing practice may be certified? ______

   ____

   ____

3. What is the national emergency telephone number? ______________

   ____

   ____

CRITICAL THINKING AND APPLICATION EXERCISES

1. Contact your local EMS to obtain information about emergency telephone numbers and response times.
2. Create a chart that compares and contrasts informed and implied consent.
3. Obtain examples of documents for advanced directives, durable power of attorney, and living wills.

CHAPTER

2

Physiologic Concepts Essential to Critical Care and Emergency Nursing

Learning objectives

After studying this chapter, you should be able to:

- Identify the core concepts essential to critical care and emergency nursing.
- Describe the regulatory mechanism used to maintain homeostasis for each concept.
- Discuss the application of each concept to critical care and emergency nursing.

Chapter overview

Caring for the patient requiring critical care and emergency nursing requires a sound understanding of the core physiologic concepts of ventilation, gas exchange, tissue perfusion, fluid and electrolyte balance, and acid-base balance. Critical care and emergency nurses base nursing activities and interventions on the core concepts and the body's regulatory mechanisms responsible for maintaining homeostasis.

♦ I. Introduction

A. Core concepts imply that common principles relate to patients in both critical care and emergency areas

B. These concepts are generalized ideas and standard elements that provide a sensible approach to mastering the principles and skills of critical care and emergency nursing

C. Core concepts are essential for rapid patient assessment and provide the foundation for nursing activities and interventions in the emergency department and critical care areas

D. Core concepts in this chapter include the following:
1. Ventilation
2. Gas exchange
3. Tissue perfusion
4. Fluid and electrolyte balance
5. Acid-base balance

E. These concepts often blend and overlap, with an imbalance in one causing an imbalance in one or more of the others

♦ II. Ventilation

A. General information
1. Ventilation is the process of moving gas into (inspiration) and out of (expiration) the lungs
2. Inspiration is an active process produced by contraction of the diaphragm and the external intercostal muscles
3. Expiration is a passive process that occurs by elastic recoil of the lungs and the chest wall
4. A negative pressure exists in the intrapleural space so that the lungs do not separate from the thorax during inspiration and expiration
5. Effective ventilation maintains a $PaCO_2$ in a healthy individual between 35 and 45 mm Hg
6. Ventilation is the initial step toward adequate gas exchange and tissue perfusion
7. As a result of disease or trauma or during the perioperative period, some patients require mechanical ventilatory support (see Chapter 7) to assist them temporarily

B. Regulation
1. Breathing is regulated by neurons in the medulla and pons, by acid-base status, and by the state of wakefulness
2. Central chemoreceptors are sensitive to changes in the carbon dioxide (CO_2) level, which is the primary stimulus for breathing

3. Peripheral chemoreceptors are sensitive to changes in the oxygen (O_2) level and in pH and provide a secondary stimulus for breathing
4. Regulation of respiratory function, including bronchiolar smooth muscle contraction or relaxation, is mainly under autonomic nervous system control

C. Application to critical care and emergency nursing
1. Patients admitted to critical care or emergency areas may have conditions that interfere with ventilation, such as airway obstruction, pulmonary embolism, or pulmonary edema
2. Ineffective ventilation leads to altered gas exchange and tissue perfusion
3. Patient care management is aimed at maintaining a patent airway and maintaining or improving ventilation
4. The ABCs (airway, breathing, and circulation) are priorities when caring for all patients

♦ III. Gas exchange

A. General information
1. Gas exchange describes two processes: the movement of O_2 from the alveoli to the bloodstream, where it is bound to hemoglobin and transported to the cells; and the movement of CO_2 from the bloodstream to the alveoli, where it is removed through exhalation
2. Adequate gas exchange requires satisfactory ventilation, perfusion, and diffusion
3. Gas exchange depends on tidal volume, the amount of air normally inhaled or exhaled; however, not all of the tidal volume reaches the alveoli, where it can participate in gas exchange
4. *Dead space* refers to the portion of tidal volume remaining in those areas that conduct air but are not involved in gas exchange; normally, this amount constitutes one-third of the tidal volume, but it may increase when physiologic dead space (areas that normally contribute to ventilation) and excessive tubing on mechanical ventilators are included
5. The tidal volume (V^T) × frequency (f) = minute ventilation (V_E)
6. Gas exchange takes place on the surface of the alveoli
7. Alveolar type II cells secrete SURFACTANT, a lipoprotein that decreases surface tension of the cell membrane and prevents alveolar collapse
8. Gas distribution to all lung areas is not uniform
9. The relationship of gas to blood flow is expressed as the ventilation-perfusion ($\dot{V}/\dot{Q}$) ratio and is normally 0.8 (4 liters/minute ventilation to 5 liters/minute perfusion)

10. When perfusion exists without ventilation, shunting occurs
    a. Blood bypasses the alveoli and does not participate in gas exchange
    b. Normally, this amounts to approximately 2% of inspired air but may be as high as 50% in certain diseases, such as adult respiratory distress syndrome
11. Insufficient O_2 exchange results in hypoxemia, and insufficient CO_2 exchange results in hypercapnia
12. The adequacy of gas exchange is determined by arterial blood gas (ABG) analysis and mixed venous blood analysis

B. Regulation
1. Gas exchange is dependent on adequate regulation of ventilation
2. Gas exchange results from diffusion based on pressure gradients across the cell membrane
3. Perfusion is regulated by cardiac output and obstruction to blood flow

C. Application to critical care and emergency nursing
1. Patients admitted to critical care or emergency areas commonly have conditions that interfere with gas exchange
2. Ineffective gas exchange leads to hypoxia, as evidenced by lactic acidosis, altered tissue perfusion, and organ dysfunction
3. Knowledge of normal and abnormal laboratory and assessment findings is essential for managing a patient with inefficient gas exchange
4. Patient care management is aimed at maintaining or improving gas exchange

♦ IV. Tissue perfusion

A. General information
1. Tissue perfusion is the process by which blood flow to the cells provides the nutrients necessary for proper cellular functioning
2. Adequate tissue perfusion is essential to adequate cellular functioning and homeostasis
3. Adequate tissue perfusion provides cells with the O_2 necessary for metabolic processes and waste removal
4. Decreased tissue perfusion decreases O_2 to the cells (tissue hypoxia), causing anaerobic metabolism and accumulation of waste products in the cells
5. These processes further result in lactic acidosis and shock

B. Regulation
1. Compensatory mechanisms are activated by inadequate tissue perfusion

2. Baroreceptors in the carotid and aortic arch stimulate the vasomotor center in the medulla
3. The sympathetic nervous system releases epinephrine and norepinephrine
4. Blood is shunted to vital organs (the heart and brain) and away from organs that tolerate ischemia (skin, skeletal muscles, and fat)
5. The respiratory rate increases to improve oxygenation
6. The renin-angiotensin-aldosterone system is activated to increase vasoconstriction and water retention
7. The posterior pituitary gland secretes antidiuretic hormone (ADH), or vasopressin, a potent vasoconstrictor, to increase water retention
   a. A shift from interstitial to vascular space of approximately 200 to 400 ml occurs

CLINICAL ALERT

   b. Compensatory mechanisms may worsen a patient's clinical condition by adding to the workload of the heart by means of increased fluid volume and vasoconstriction

C. Application to critical care and emergency nursing
1. Patients admitted to critical care or emergency areas typically have conditions that adversely affect tissue perfusion
2. As abnormal tissue perfusion occurs, shock develops, causing alterations in tissue metabolism and death of tissue cells
3. Accurate assessment of tissue perfusion and prompt intervention can improve the patient's chances for survival

♦ V. Fluid and electrolyte balance

A. General information
1. Fluid and electrolyte balance describes the body's normal ratio of water to ELECTROLYTES within body fluids
2. Water in the body carries nutrients and waste material and is expressed as a percentage of body weight
3. The amount of water in the body is related to age, gender, and body fat; in adults, water content is 60% of body weight in the average man and 50% in the average woman; older adults have a lower percentage of body water, and children have a higher percentage
4. Body water is distributed between two major fluid compartments: extracellular and intracellular
5. *Extracellular fluid* (ECF) constitutes one-third of total body water and is found in the blood vessels as plasma and between the cells as interstitial fluid
6. *Intracellular fluid* (ICF) constitutes two-thirds of total body water and is found within the cell

7. Electrolytes are positively or negatively charged substances that unite in various combinations in body fluids and differ in concentration in ECF and ICF
8. Major ECF electrolytes include sodium (Na^+, the principal cation), chloride (Cl^+), and bicarbonate (HCO_3^-)
9. Major ICF electrolytes include potassium (K^+), magnesium (Mg^{++}), phosphates, and proteins
10. Fluid (water and electrolytes) moves between compartments; fluid movement is determined by the permeability of the membrane separating the fluid compartments, fluid osmolality, ECF concentration of Na^+, crystalloid and COLLOIDAL OSMOTIC PRESSURE, and CAPILLARY HYDROSTATIC PRESSURE
11. Mechanisms by which water and electrolytes move between fluid compartments include DIFFUSION, OSMOSIS, and active transport (sodium-potassium pump)

B. Regulation

1. Compensatory mechanisms maintain fluid and electrolyte levels within normal range
2. For homeostasis to occur, fluid intake must equal fluid output; average daily fluid intake is approximately 2,600 ml; average daily fluid output is 2,600 ml, which includes water lost as urine, in stool, and through the lungs and skin
3. Specific organs and glands also help to regulate fluid and electrolyte balance
4. Kidneys perform major regulatory functions, including retention and excretion of fluids and select electrolytes, regulation of pH and excretion of metabolic waste and toxic substances, and secretion of renin as a response to decreased blood pressure or ECF volume
5. Through its pumping action, the heart maintains the kidneys' perfusion pressure to regulate water and electrolyte balance
6. The lungs maintain acid-base balance and contribute to insensible water loss; renin interacts with angiotensinogen in the liver to form angiotensin I, which converts to angiotensin II, a potent vasopressor, in the lungs
7. The adrenal glands secrete aldosterone, which alters the fluid balance
   a. Increased aldosterone secretion retains Na^+, increasing water retention and K^+ loss
   b. Decreased aldosterone secretion causes Na^+ and water loss and K^+ retention
   c. Angiotensin II stimulates the production and secretion of aldosterone

8. The hypothalamus responds to increased serum osmolality, which stimulates the thirst center and the need for water ingestion; it also produces ADH
9. The posterior pituitary gland secretes ADH, causing fluid retention
   a. The primary stimulus for secretion is increased serum osmolality
   b. The secondary stimulus is a severe ECF deficit
10. The parathyroid glands regulate calcium and phosphate by secreting parathyroid hormone, which affects bone resorption and calcium absorption and reabsorption

C. Application to critical care and emergency nursing
1. Healthy people can cope with changes in fluid and electrolyte composition
2. Patients admitted to critical care or emergency areas typically suffer from conditions that alter their fluid and electrolyte balance or restrict their ability to eat and drink to maintain an equilibrium in fluids and electrolytes
3. Patients experience various changes that disrupt physiologic and psychological integrity because of fluid and electrolyte imbalances
4. Patient care management is aimed at restoring and maintaining fluid and electrolyte balance

♦ VI. Acid-base balance

A. General information
1. The normal ratio of acid to base is 1:20, representing one part acid, such as CO_2, to 20 parts base, such as HCO_3^-
2. Metabolic processes must maintain a steady balance of acids and bases to ensure optimum cellular functioning
3. An acid is any substance that can donate or give up hydrogen ions (H^+)
4. A base is any substance that can accept H^+
5. Acid-base balance is measured by ABG analysis (see *Normal ABG values*)
6. Arterial blood pH is an indirect measurement of H^+ concentration
7. Arterial blood carbon dioxide ($Paco_2$) measures the partial pressure of CO_2 in arterial blood
   a. It reflects alveolar ventilation
   b. It is the respiratory component of acid-base balance
8. Arterial blood bicarbonate (HCO_3^-) reflects the metabolic component of acid-base balance
9. Arterial blood oxygen (Pao_2) measures the partial pressure of O_2 in arterial blood and reflects the adequacy of oxygenation
10. Arterial blood oxygen saturation measures the percentage of hemoglobin saturated with O_2

Normal ABG values

pH	7.35 to 7.45
$PaCO_2$	35 to 45 mm Hg
HCO_3^-	22 to 26 mEq/liter
PaO_2	80 to 100 mm Hg
SaO_2	95% to 100%
Base excess	-2.5 to +2.5

CLINICAL ALERT

11. Arterial blood base excess reflects the amount of buffering present
12. Body temperature and O_2 content of inspired air must be determined for accurate ABG analysis

B. Regulation
1. Acids are continuously liberated as metabolic by-products
2. Body buffer systems prevent large changes in pH by chemically combining acids with other ions
3. The respiratory system is responsible for regulating the body's CO_2 level; the renal system is responsible for regulating the body's HCO_3^- level
4. Compensation occurs as a response by the system not primarily affected to minimize changes in pH or to return pH to near normal
   a. Respiratory imbalances result in metabolic compensation by the kidneys, which may take several days
   b. Metabolic imbalances result in respiratory compensation by the lungs, which begins within minutes

CLINICAL ALERT

   c. Patients with conditions that affect the lungs or kidneys may be unable to compensate for imbalances
5. Correction of acid-base imbalances to return the pH to normal depends on a physiologic or therapeutic response by the system primarily affected

C. Application to critical care and emergency nursing
1. Patients admitted to critical care or emergency areas typically have conditions that alter acid-base balance
2. Patients with acid-base imbalances experience various changes that disrupt overall body functioning
3. Knowledge of acid-base balance, compensation, and correction is crucial to promote optimum body functioning

4. Knowledge of normal and abnormal ABG values indicating acid-base balance or imbalance is essential for effective patient care management
5. Patient care management is aimed at restoring and maintaining acid-base balance

Points to remember

- Adequate tissue perfusion is essential to adequate cellular functioning.
- Changes in the CO_2 level are the primary stimulus for breathing.
- O_2 is transported in the blood primarily by binding with hemoglobin.
- A steady balance (1:20) between acids and bases must be maintained for optimum cellular functioning.
- Arterial blood pH is an indirect measurement of the H^+ concentration.
- Fluid movement is determined by cell membrane permeability, fluid osmolality, crystalloid and colloid osmotic pressure, and capillary hydrostatic pressure.

Study questions

To evaluate your understanding of this chapter, answer the following questions in the space provided; then compare your responses with the correct answers in Appendix B, page 279.

1. What are the normal ABG values? 7.35-7.45 pH
   pCO2 - 35-45
   pHCO3- 22-26 PO2 90-100

2. Which major regulatory functions of the kidneys are used to regulate fluid and electrolyte balance? retention & excretion of fluids + electrolytes Regulation of pH metabolites waste excretion + renin excretion

3. Which key compensatory mechanisms are activated by inadequate tissue perfusion? renin-angiotensin-aldosterone ADH, lactic acid release

4. Where does gas exchange take place in the lungs? aveoli

CRITICAL THINKING AND APPLICATION EXERCISES

1. Analyze a set of your patient's blood gases in relation to oxygenation and acid-base balance, and relate the results to the patient's clinical condition.
2. Discuss why a patient with emphysema would be at risk for problems with gas exchange.
3. Prepare an oral class presentation on why the ABGs of a patient in cardio-pulmonary arrest would show respiratory and metabolic acidosis.
4. Explain why a patient with a brain tumor affecting his medulla would be at risk for altered breathing patterns.

CHAPTER

3

Psychosocial Aspects of Critical Care and Emergency Nursing

Learning objectives

After studying this chapter, you should be able to:

- Identify the general principles related to the psychosocial implications of critical and emergency illness.
- Name major problems that confront the patient and family during critical or emergency illness or hospitalization.
- Discuss common physical and behavioral assessment findings for the patient with impaired psychosocial integrity.
- Describe patient care management for the patient and family in crisis because of illness or hospitalization.

Chapter overview

Physiologic injury or illness is only one component in the management of patients in critical care or emergency areas. The dynamic nature of the cycle of health and illness and the factors that affect the patient's basic coping mechanisms impact on recovery and the patient's and family's response to crisis. Nursing care focuses on physical and behavioral assessment findings for the patient with impaired psychosocial integrity and on measures to assist the patient and family in crisis.

♦ I. Introduction

A. Cycle of health and illness
   1. Most patients go through three stages
      a. A transition from health to illness, at which time the patient and family experience denial, disbelief, or shock
      b. A developing awareness and acceptance that the patient needs help from others
      c. A reorganizational period in which the patient's interest in life is renewed and he or she makes plans for the future
   2. These stages are dynamic; patients may move from one stage to another, depending on the stressors and how they affect coping mechanisms

B. Factors affecting coping response
   1. Critical or emergency illness alters a patient's sense of well-being, independence, and self-esteem as he or she faces the task of coping with the illness
   2. The patient and family try to adapt to critical or emergency illness by using coping skills that differ in appropriateness and helpfulness
   3. Most patients use previously employed coping patterns, either consciously or unconsciously, to deal with the environment and their situation
   4. Factors that affect the patient's basic coping mechanisms result from exposure to stressors
   5. Individual stressors do not affect everyone equally
      a. Biologic stressors include an injury or illness, its severity, and the patient's perception of its significance
      b. Psychosocial stressors include interpersonal conflicts with family members, legal or financial considerations, and growth and developmental conflicts
      c. Environmental stressors in the emergency department (ED) or intensive care unit (ICU) include unfamiliarity with the surroundings, sensory overload, sensory deprivation, limited family visitation, and isolation

C. Psychosocial problems
   1. Patients in the ED or ICU experience psychosocial problems from FEAR, depression, POWERLESSNESS, sleep deprivation, or ANXIETY
   2. Patients commonly have difficulty communicating their fears, anxiety, or pain; such difficulty aggravates their already compromised state

CLINICAL ALERT

   3. Patients and their families commonly are unsettled and frightened by the overwhelming critical care and emergency environments

D. Patient needs and responses
1. Admission to an ED, and particularly to an ICU, severely disrupts the patient's and family's routine; different surroundings, rules, smells, and people cause stress on the patient's territorial needs
2. The territorial needs of privacy, autonomy, self-identity, and security must be met; to do so in a hospital, the patient establishes a temporary territory
3. When TERRITORIALITY is overlooked by the nurse, the patient's feeling of lack of control may lead to anxiety
4. Signs of anxiety in the patient or family depend on the degree of anxiety experienced
   a. Mild anxiety can heighten the use of coping skills
   b. Severe anxiety can incapacitate the patient
5. Patients and families face major problems during illness, which may occur simultaneously with or recur periodically during the illness
   a. Dealing with the symptoms, discomfort, and incapacitation of the illness or injury
   b. Managing the stress of treatments and hospitalization
   c. Developing and maintaining relationships with members of the medical team
   d. Maintaining a positive self-image and a sense of competence
   e. Dealing with the disturbing feelings evoked by illness or treatment
   f. Maintaining relationships with family and significant others despite role alterations
   g. Preparing for an uncertain future
6. During critical or emergency illness, many patients search for wholeness, spirituality, and ways to create new perceptions for their lives

CLINICAL ALERT

7. The universal need of families in crisis is hope; effective communication among the patient, family, and nurse is essential and can help reduce anxiety, identify health needs, clarify misconceptions, and develop a supportive relationship
8. Emotional response coupled with the increased sympathetic nervous system response increases myocardial oxygen consumption; it is important for the nurse to help mediate this response to minimize possible tissue damage resulting from hypoxia

♦ II. Assessing the need for psychosocial intervention

A. Physical assessment findings
1. Increased muscle tension
2. Increased perspiration, clammy skin
3. Fatigue
4. Restlessness
5. Increased heart rate

6. Increased rate or depth of respiration
7. Diarrhea
8. Urinary urgency
9. Decreased appetite
10. Dilated pupils
11. Changes in body temperature or blood pressure

B. Behavioral assessment findings
1. Increased number of questions
2. Increased verbalization of anxiety
3. Increased focus on equipment or procedures
4. Increased acting out
5. Decreased focus on feelings
6. Decreased ability to follow directions

♦ III. Patient care management

A. Goals
1. Resolve the immediate problem
2. Regain equilibrium
3. Resolve the overall crisis

B. Possible nursing diagnoses for a patient in crisis because of illness, injury, or hospitalization
1. Anxiety
2. Ineffective individual coping
3. Altered role performance
4. Fear
5. Spiritual distress
6. Impaired social interaction
7. Sensory or perceptual alterations
8. Ineffective family coping: compromised
9. Altered family processes
10. Hopelessness
11. Powerlessness

C. Strategies
1. Orient the patient and family to the environment to alleviate anxiety
2. Explain nursing actions and treatment (for specific teaching tips, see *Dealing with critical or emergency illness,* page 22)
3. Give the patient personal and environmental control alternatives to alleviate feelings of powerlessness
4. Include family or support people in explanations and care
5. Maintain appropriate wake and sleep cycles to encourage normal sleep patterns
6. Minimize conversation and equipment noise to prevent sensory overload

TEACHING TIPS

Dealing with critical or emergency illness

Be sure to include the following topics in your teaching plan for the patient and family in crisis.

- Previous and current coping behaviors
- Strengths and positive coping behaviors
- Identification and reduction of stressors
- Effective interaction with others
- Self-care activities
- Expression of appropriate concern for medical condition
- Active participation in decisions regarding care, treatment, and the future
- Self-regulating interventions (such as relaxation, imagery, and music therapy) to balance the patient's response to illness

7. Provide information the patient needs to be effective in a given situation
8. Provide opportunities for private interactions between the patient and family
9. Recognize that people differ in their ability to use strategies effectively
10. Assist the family in understanding that the patient may use anger, denial, and increased dependency in early stages of crisis as adaptive coping behaviors until effective coping responses are acquired
11. Recognize that many patients and families find comfort in religion and prayer; a visit from their minister or the hospital chaplain can provide positive support

CLINICAL ALERT

12. Be aware that the needs of the patient and family may change over time; continually reassess to plan appropriate interventions

POINTS TO REMEMBER

- Critical care and emergency nurses need to recognize anxiety and encourage the patient and family to express concerns and fears.
- Most people use previously employed coping mechanisms to deal with a changed environment and an unfamiliar situation.
- Denial, anger, withdrawal, and demanding behavior may reflect coping patterns used during critical and emergency illnesses.
- Critical or emergency illness is a potential life crisis for the patient and family.

Study Questions

To evaluate your understanding of this chapter, answer the following questions in the space provided; then compare your responses with the correct answers in Appendix B, pages 279 and 280.

1. Which three stages does the patient experience in the cycle of health and illness? ______________________________

2. Which stressors affect a patient's basic coping mechanisms? ______________________________

3. Which self-regulating interventions may help patients balance their response to illness? ______________________________

Critical Thinking and Application Exercises

1. Interview family members of a patient in a critical care area and discuss their priority concerns.
2. Follow a patient through his ED experience, and assess the basic coping mechanisms present.
3. Discuss with a hospital chaplain or local minister the role that spirituality and religion play during critical or emergency illness, injury, or hospitalization.
4. With a group of fellow students, discuss which fears you would have if you developed a critical or an emergency illness or injury.

CHAPTER

4

Nutritional Support

Learning objectives

After studying this chapter, you should be able to:

- Describe the general principles related to nutritional support.
- Identify physiologic changes caused by inadequate nutrition.
- Discuss the common physical assessment and diagnostic test findings related to inadequate nutrition.
- Describe care management for the patient receiving nutritional support.

Chapter overview

Adequate nutrition is especially important for patients in critical care and emergency areas because they are vulnerable to the stress of injury or illness. Metabolic requirements depend on basal metabolic needs, activity, growth, health status, and stress. Assessment of nutritional status involves evaluation of data regarding diet and medical history, physical examination, and laboratory data. Inadequate nutrition leads to physiologic changes that may require either enteral or parenteral nutritional support. The goals of patient care management are to maintain lean body mass and to provide adequate nutrients and energy to sustain physiologic processes. Many strategies are used to ensure that these goals are met.

♦ I. Introduction

A. Nutrient needs
   1. Adequate nutrition exists when carbohydrates, proteins, fats, water, vitamins, and minerals are consumed in sufficient amounts to meet the body's metabolic requirements
   2. The amount of nutrients needed to meet metabolic requirements is based on changes related to basal metabolic needs, activity, growth, health status, and stress
   3. Without a supply of dextrose, serum insulin levels drop, causing body fat to be used as energy; free fatty acids are mobilized from adipose tissue and are broken down in the liver to ketone bodies, causing KETOSIS
   4. Inadequate nutrition causes the progressive loss of lean body mass and fat stores as the body's demands exceed its intake; this can lead to impaired wound healing, decreased resistance to infection, muscle wasting, inefficient cell-mediated immunity, pressure ulcer formation, anemia, and death

B. Risk factors for inadequate nutrition
   1. Age (infants, children, older adults)
   2. Recent illness or injury
   3. History of alcohol or drug abuse
   4. Severe trauma
   5. Serious infection
   6. Prolonged fever
   7. Massive burns
   8. Prolonged nausea, vomiting, diarrhea
   9. Wound drainage or dialysis
   10. Decreased GI tract perfusion

C. Indicators of nutritional status
   1. History
   2. Physical examination
      a. Quality of wound healing
      b. Appearance of skin and hair
      c. Degree of muscle wasting
      d. Body weight

CLINICAL ALERT

         (1) Body weight is a less reliable indicator of nutritional status in a patient with an unstable volume status
         (2) Interpretation of weight trends in patients with unstable volume status may be difficult but must include intracellular fluid shifts, extracellular fluid shifts, diuresis, and weight of dressing or equipment

3. Laboratory data
   a. Serum proteins
   b. Hemoglobin and hematocrit
   c. Nitrogen balance
   d. Urine creatinine

♦ II. Nutritional support

A. General information
1. Critically ill patients are at high risk for developing malnutrition because of conditions that limit intake or nutrient absorption or that increase nutritional demands
2. Many critically ill patients cannot meet nutritional requirements orally

CLINICAL ALERT

3. Illness, injury, and trauma create a physiologic stress that increases the metabolic rate, causing increased oxygen consumption and energy expenditure

B. Formula selection
1. The nutritional support formula chosen and the route of administration depend on nutritional needs, fluid tolerance, and absorptive abilities of the GI tract
2. The choice of nutritional support formula is based on its OSMOLALITY (the concentration of carbohydrates, amino acids, and electrolytes determines the osmolality of nutritional formulas)
   a. Isotonic solutions have about the same osmolality as blood (300 mOsm)
   b. Hypertonic or hyperosmolar solutions have a greater osmolality than blood

C. Routes
1. Nutrients must be given in a form that is nutritionally acceptable, tolerated, and utilized
2. Alternate methods of feeding can be used
   a. Tube or enteral feedings
   b. Peripheral I.V. infusion
   c. Peripheral parenteral nutrition (PPN), which delivers nutrition through peripheral veins
   d. Total parenteral nutrition (TPN), which delivers nutrition through a central vein
   e. Parenteral lipid emulsions

D. Enteral feedings
1. Enteral feedings are used for patients who have some digestive and absorptive function but are unable or unwilling to consume food by mouth in sufficient quantities to meet caloric requirements

2. Enteral nutritional support given by the nasogastric, gastric, or jejunostomy route usually involves commercially prepared formulas
   a. Iso-osmolar: providing approximately 1 calorie/ml; has the same osmolality as plasma
   b. Hyperosmolar: providing approximately 1 to 2 calories/ml; high osmolality makes this type of formula less well tolerated
   c. Elemental: providing specific nutrient components with high osmolality; best tolerated if administered into the small bowel
   d. Special formulas: restricting protein, sodium, or potassium; given to patients with kidney or liver disease
3. Enteral feedings may be administered by the continuous-drip method or by intermittent bolus feedings
4. Enteral feedings administered too rapidly or before the patient has adjusted to the high concentration of particles can cause water to rush into the intestine and dilute the particles in concentration, which can lead to nausea, cramping, and diarrhea (dumping syndrome)

E. Parenteral feedings
1. Parenteral nutrition is indicated in patients who are unable to ingest or absorb adequate nutrients by way of the GI tract
2. Parenteral nutrition is given through a peripheral or central I.V. line
   a. Peripheral I.V. solutions consist of water with glucose, electrolytes, or both; they are used short term because they have little nutritional or caloric value
   b. PPN solutions are administered through a peripheral I.V. line
      (1) They consist of an isotonic or a hypotonic infusion of dextrose (5% to 10%), amino acids (3% to 8.5%), vitamins, electrolytes, and trace elements
      (2) They provide temporary nutritional support to promote nitrogen balance and weight gain when the enteral route is inadequate or contraindicated or during transition from TPN to enteral intake
   c. TPN solutions are administered through a central I.V. line
      (1) They consist of a hypertonic complete nutrition solution of dextrose (25% to 70%), amino acids (3.5% to 10%), vitamins, electrolytes, and trace elements
      (2) Their composition depends on the patient's nutritional needs and clinical condition
      (3) They provide complete nutritional support when the enteral route is inadequate or contraindicated
   d. Parenteral lipid emulsions consist of essential fatty acids (10% or 20%)

(1) Isotonic fat emulsion can contribute up to 60% of the total daily caloric intake to correct or prevent essential fatty acid deficiency

(2) These emulsions are usually recommended in combination with TPN or PPN but can be used by themselves to replace carbohydrate calories in patients with glucose intolerance or when carbon dioxide (CO_2) production must be avoided

♦ III. Assessing the need for nutritional support

A. Physical assessment findings

1. Recent unplanned weight loss equaling 10% or more of normal weight
2. Anthropometric measurement: triceps skin-fold and mid-upper-arm muscle circumference measurements less than standard
3. Tissue wasting
4. Hair loss
5. Delayed wound healing
6. Petechiae or ecchymoses

B. Diagnostic test findings

1. Nitrogen balance: negative
2. Serum albumin levels: less than 4 grams/dl
3. Serum transferrin levels: less than 250 mcg/dl
4. Hemoglobin levels: less than 12 grams/dl (female); less than 14 grams/dl (male)
5. Hematocrit levels: less than 37% (female); less than 45% (male)
6. Total protein levels: less than 6 grams/dl
7. Urine urea nitrogen levels: increased nitrogen (in early inadequate nutritional states); decreased nitrogen (in late inadequate nutritional states)

♦ IV. Patient care management for enteral nutrition

A. Goals

1. Maintain lean body mass
2. Provide adequate nutrients and energy to sustain physiologic processes

B. Potential nursing diagnoses for the patient who needs nutritional support

1. Altered nutrition: less than body requirements
2. Risk for infection
3. Impaired skin integrity

C. Strategies

1. Perform a nutritional assessment

   a. Monitor serum diagnostic tests for abnormalities
   b. Obtain triceps skin-fold and mid-upper-arm muscle measurements and compare with standards; measurements are typically difficult to obtain in critically ill patients
   c. Perform a 24-hour dietary recall and calorie counts
2. Assess the placement and function of the feeding tube
   a. Check the position of the large-bore tube by injecting air while listening over the stomach with a stethoscope or by aspirating gastric contents
   b. Do not initiate tube feeding through a small-bore tube until the tube's position has been documented by X-ray
3. Assess for intolerance to formula, as evidenced by stool frequency and consistency, nausea or vomiting, GASTRIC RESIDUAL, and abdominal distention
4. Raise the head of the bed 30 degrees, if possible, to enhance gravity flow; maintain this position for 1 hour after feeding to decrease risk of reflux and aspiration
5. Check the gastric residual by aspirating stomach contents
   a. If the residual is greater than 100 ml, return the aspirate and notify the doctor, or follow institutional policy on continuation of feeding
   b. If the residual is less than 100 ml, return the aspirate and continue feeding
6. Assess fluid and hydration status
   a. Record input and output (I/O), assessing 24-hour trends
   b. Weigh the patient daily at the same time with the same scale and with the same amount of linens or clothes
7. Monitor for diarrhea, which may be caused by problems with the formula administration
   a. If the feeding rate is too fast, start feeding at 50 ml/hour and increase by 25 ml/hour every 8 to 12 hours, depending on the patient's tolerance or the doctor's order
   b. If the formula volume is too great, decrease it to a level tolerated by the patient, gradually increasing it as tolerated; feed smaller volumes at more frequent intervals or use a continuous-drip method of administration
   c. If the formula is too cold, administer it at room temperature
   d. Give initial feeding of hypertonic formula at one-third to one-half the rate for a minimum of 8 hours, gradually increasing the concentration; do not increase rate and strength at the same time
   e. If the patient has a low serum albumin level (decreased oncotic pressure causes increased water in the bowel, leading to diar-

CLINICAL ALERT

rhea), consider diluting the formula and increasing the concentration gradually

f. Be aware that sorbitol in liquid medications may contribute to much of the diarrhea attributed to tube feedings

8. Institute measures to prevent bacterial contamination of the formula and equipment
   a. Wash hands before handling equipment
   b. Administer the formula promptly after opening; do not add newly opened formula to formula in the bag
   c. Replace the feeding bag and tubing according to institutional policy
   d. Cover and date the unused formula and store it in the refrigerator; use it within 24 hours or as recommended by manufacturer
   e. Do not allow continuous-drip solutions to hang longer than 8 hours
   f. Rinse equipment before and after feeding
9. Assess the patient for regurgitation of stomach contents, leading to potential aspiration pneumonia
   a. Elevate the head of the bed 30 degrees for at least 1 hour after feeding to ensure proper feeding position
   b. If the patient experiences slowed gastric emptying time (gastric residual greater than 100 ml), check the gastric residual before each intermittent feeding and every 4 hours with the continuous-drip method
   c. If the gastroesophageal sphincter becomes incompetent from the large-bore feeding tube, change to a feeding tube with a smaller diameter
   d. Check the tube position every shift to prevent improper placement
10. Assess for complaints of nausea
    a. Explain the procedure to the patient to allay anxiety, and provide time for questions and emotional support
    b. Check the tube for proper placement
    c. Decrease the rate of feeding or use the continuous-drip method if the feeding rate is too rapid
    d. If the volume is too great or gastric emptying is delayed, reduce the rate and then increase it gradually; check the gastric residual, and if greater than 100 ml, replace aspirated residual and follow institutional policy; encourage ambulation if distention is a problem
    e. Notify the doctor of any intolerance to a specific formula so that he can consider changing to another formula
11. Assess for possible fluid volume imbalances

TEACHING TIPS

Home enteral nutrition

Be sure to include the following topics in your teaching plan for the patient requiring tube feedings.

- Rationale for tube feeding
- Hand-washing and infection-control measures
- Procedure for carrying out the feeding
- Care of tube and equipment, including storage of solutions and temperatures for administration
- Assessment of tube placement
- Proper patient positioning for feeding
- Tube flushing after administering medications through the tube
- Ways to make the patient's environment as pleasant as possible during feeding
- Signs and symptoms of intolerance or complications and the need for notifying the doctor
- Medical follow-up

a. Assess trends in I/O, checking for alternate reasons for fluid gain or loss

b. Check for excess water entering the feeding tube either from rinsing the tube or from administering the medication

c. Monitor for excessive protein intake, which can increase urine output; evaluate the patient's protein requirements, increasing fluid intake, if possible

12. Maintain feeding tube patency

a. Flush the tube before and after each feeding with 30 to 50 ml of water

CLINICAL ALERT

b. Have the pharmacy prepare medications so they can be properly administered by way of the tube

c. Know that some medications should not be crushed

d. Note that a small-bore feeding tube may not deliver high-viscosity formulas efficiently; instead, infuse these formulas by pump or notify the doctor so he can consider low-viscosity formulas

13. Instruct the patient and family about enteral feedings if they are to be continued at home (for specific teaching tips, see *Home enteral nutrition*)

♦ V. Patient care management for parenteral nutrition

A. Goals

1. Maintain lean body mass
2. Provide adequate nutrients and energy to sustain physiologic processes

B. Possible nursing diagnoses for the patient who needs parenteral nutrition

1. Altered nutrition: less than body requirements
2. Risk for infection
3. Impaired skin integrity

C. Strategies

1. Perform a nutritional assessment
   a. Obtain serum diagnostic tests for abnormalities
   b. Assess triceps skin-fold and mid-upper-arm muscle measurements and compare with standards
   c. Perform a 24-hour dietary recall and calorie counts
   d. Obtain the patient's weight and compare it with baseline
   e. Estimate nonprotein caloric needs by using calorimetry and the HARRIS-BENEDICT EQUATION
2. Maintain aseptic technique, using thorough hand washing before touching to prevent infection
3. Record I/O, assessing 24-hour trends to prevent fluid imbalances
4. Control infusion rate with an I.V. pump to prevent fluid overload
5. Observe for complications of TPN, including sepsis, line occlusion, glucose intolerance, and fungal infection
6. Minimize the risk of infection for a patient receiving TPN
   a. Do not use the TPN line to give blood, administer medications, or measure central venous pressure
   b. Allow the TPN solution to hang for no longer than 24 hours; use a filter to prevent infusion of gross particles
   c. Keep the TPN solution refrigerated until administration, and check the label on fluids for correct name and concentrations
   d. Change the catheter and dressing according to institutional policy
7. Monitor fluid and electrolyte levels to prevent possible imbalances
   a. Start the infusion rate slowly to allow the patient's body to adapt to the high glucose load and osmolality; gradually increase the rate, as ordered, until the desired rate is achieved
   b. If the infusion falls behind, do not attempt to compensate by adjusting it to a higher-than-desired rate; hyperosmolar diuresis may result from excessive glucose infusion
   c. Gradually wean the patient from TPN to prevent rebound hypoglycemia; use a dextrose 10% solution temporarily if replacement TPN solution is not readily available from the pharmacy

CLINICAL ALERT

   d. Monitor serum electrolyte levels to prevent imbalances; obtain fingerstick blood glucose levels to detect hyperglycemia
   e. Remember that the end product of carbohydrate metabolism is CO_2, which may increase $PaCO_2$ levels in patients with respiratory compromise

8. Administer lipid emulsions, as ordered, to correct fatty acid deficiency
   a. Do not give I.V. lipids to patients with abnormal lipid metabolism, severe liver disease, or acute pancreatitis
   b. Check the manufacturer's directions for lipid emulsion storage; let refrigerated emulsion stand at room temperature for 30 minutes before hanging
   c. Do not shake fat emulsions to prevent separation
   d. Hang the fat emulsion with the TPN solution, according to institutional policy, connected beyond the filter and as close to the insertion site as possible

POINTS TO REMEMBER

- Critically ill patients are at high risk for inadequate nutrition from conditions that increase nutritional demands or limit nutrient intake or absorption.
- Enteral feedings may be administered by the continuous-drip method or by intermittent bolus feedings.
- Complications associated with TPN include sepsis, glucose intolerance, line occlusion, and fungal infection.

STUDY QUESTIONS

To evaluate your understanding of this chapter, answer the following questions in the space provided; then compare your responses with the correct answers in Appendix B, page 280.

1. Which alternate feeding methods are available to provide nutritional support to the critically ill and emergency patient? ______________________

   ____

   ____

2. How does one assess for placement of a nasogastric tube? ______________

   ____

   ____

3. Which nursing actions minimize the risk of infection for a patient receiving TPN? ____

____

____

CRITICAL THINKING AND APPLICATION EXERCISES

1. Perform a nutritional assessment on a patient, and identify the areas of risk.
2. Compare and contrast the variations in nutritional interventions in a patient with a cardiovascular disorder and a patient with a renal disorder.
3. Describe the additional nutritional problems encountered by a patient who is already undernourished when faced with a critical illness.
4. Obtain a nutritional history from a fellow student. Evaluate the information and develop a teaching plan.

CHAPTER

5

Infection Control

Learning objectives

After studying this chapter, you should be able to:

- Describe the general principles related to infection control.
- Identify the common causes of infection in the critically ill patient.
- Discuss the common physical assessment and diagnostic test findings used to determine the need for infection control.
- Describe care management for the patient with an infection.

Chapter overview

Critically ill patients are commonly immunocompromised or debilitated. Along with very young and elderly patients, they are at greatest risk for infection. Hand washing is the primary means of preventing the spread of infection. Prophylactic antibiotic therapy and abuse of antibiotics have contributed to the development of resistant microorganisms. Aseptic technique, proper identification of causative organisms, and specific drug therapy are essential to preventing and treating the spread of infection.

I. Basic concepts

A. Infection prevention

1. Although all patients must be protected from infection, patients with active infections are most in need of infection-control measures
2. Critically ill patients are at grave risk for infection because their immune systems are commonly debilitated and severely compromised
3. Certain disease processes, such as diabetes, severe trauma, renal failure, chronic lung disease, and leukemia, predispose the patient to an increased risk for infection
4. A patient being treated for one infection may develop a secondary infection from exposure in the hospital or from antibiotic therapy

B. Common causes of infection

1. The most common cause of SEPTICEMIA is the insertion of intravascular devices
   a. Critically ill patients typically require the placement of central or peripheral vascular access lines for hemodynamic monitoring
   b. Bacteremia acquired in the critical care unit usually originates from the insertion of intravascular catheters
2. Antibiotic-RESISTANT ORGANISMS are a major cause of infection in critically ill patients
   a. Infection results from liberal use of broad-spectrum antibiotics
   b. The most common organisms include staphylococci, Enterobacteriaceae, Pseudomonas, Candida, tuberculosis, enterococcus, and streptococci

C. Common infection sites

CLINICAL ALERT

1. The most common infection sites in the critically ill patient are the urinary tract, the respiratory tract, the wound site, and the blood
2. Approximately 50% of the patients who acquire septicemia die as a result; it can occur in patients of all ages and in acutely and chronically ill patients

D. Infection control

1. The Centers for Disease Control and Prevention (CDC) has recommended the use of Standard Precautions as the minimal level of precautions for all patients receiving care in hospitals (Refer to current CDC guidelines.)
2. Infection is a risk because the patient admitted on an emergency basis may be unable to communicate previous exposure to or presence of infectious disease
3. Concern over life-threatening illness may take precedence over suspected infectious disease

♦ II. Assessing the need for infection control

A. Physical assessment findings

1. Symptoms may be masked or absent if the patient is immunosuppressed or receiving antibiotics
2. Local symptoms depend on the infection site and may include edema, inflammation, redness, elevated temperature, and purulent drainage
3. Systemic symptoms may include fever, chills, and tachycardia

B. Diagnostic test findings

1. White blood cell (WBC) count is elevated unless the causative organism is viral or mycoplasmic
2. WBC differential assists in differentiating the type of infection (for example, an increase in neutrophils is evidence that the body is fighting a bacterial infection)
3. Culture and sensitivity studies identify the organism and reveal the appropriate antibiotic to use for treatment

CLINICAL ALERT

4. About 50% of the patients with septicemia do not have a positive culture returned

♦ III. Patient care management

A. Goals

1. Identify the patient at risk
2. Prevent the spread of infection
3. Treat the identified infection

B. Possible nursing diagnoses for a patient with an infection

1. Altered tissue perfusion
2. Social isolation
3. Knowledge deficit

C. Strategies

1. Obtain diagnostic studies to identify the source of the infection
   a. Diagnostic studies are valid only if the specimen is properly collected, transported, and processed
   b. Collection protocols may vary among institutions
   c. To prevent contamination, use strict sterile technique when collecting a specimen to be studied for culture
2. Administer drugs, as ordered
   a. Antibiotics appropriate to the organism are given at specified times, according to pharmacologic recommendations for the presence or absence of food in the gut, to maintain adequate blood levels
   b. Evaluation of the patient's kidney and liver function is essential to determine the correct dosage

c. Resistant organisms may require frequent adjustments in choice and dosage of drugs
d. Appropriate drugs treat the underlying pathophysiologic process contributing to the infection; these include insulin for diabetes and bronchodilators for chronic lung disease

3. Follow CDC Standard Precautions; wear gloves any time skin or mucous membrane is likely to contact blood or other body fluids; wear a protective apron or mask as necessary
   a. Procedures likely to cause contamination from excreta include suctioning, dressing changes, urine measurement, toileting, and blood specimen collection
   b. Precautions protect the patient and the nurse
4. Wash hands, using vigorous friction, under running water with standard soap for a minimum of 10 seconds; this is the primary means of preventing infection transmission
   a. Antiseptic soaps and a longer washing time should be used in high-risk clinical areas and for invasive procedures (may vary according to institutional policy)
   b. Hands should be washed between contact with different patients, between different procedures on the same patient, and before and after gloves are worn (skin flora multiply rapidly in gloves)
5. Adhere strictly to protocols for catheter insertion and care to markedly reduce CATHETER-RELATED SEPSIS
   a. Use of any catheter (urinary or vascular) must be essential for care, not merely a convenience for the medical or nursing staff
   b. Any catheter must be inserted under strict sterile conditions
   c. Site care must be performed according to CDC guidelines and institutional policy
   d. All connection sites are potential sources of contamination; the catheter system should be manipulated only after strict hand washing or glove donning
6. Decrease risks of infection by adhering to established guidelines
   a. Sharing of equipment between patients should be avoided to prevent CROSS-CONTAMINATION
   b. Equipment needing careful decontamination includes that which cannot be autoclaved, such as transducers, monitor parts, and oxygen and ventilator equipment
   c. Spills, especially blood and other excreta, should be removed immediately
   d. Personnel with active infections, especially upper respiratory tract infections and herpetic lesions, should be restricted from patient contact

TEACHING TIPS
Infection control

Be sure to include the following topics in your teaching plan for the patient when discussing infection control.

- Risk factors and causative agents contributing to the infection
- Specific drug regimens for treatment
- Importance of informing others of infection if it will have a major health effect, such as with hepatitis, herpes, or acquired immunodeficiency syndrome
- Hand-washing techniques and frequency
- Specific measures to prevent and control infection
- Proper disposal of contaminated materials

7. Care for infection sites properly
   a. Dressings should be changed as frequently as necessary to keep the site clean and dry
   b. Cross-contamination of sites is prevented by covering each area with a separate dressing
   c. Wound care varies according to site, infective organism, and institutional policy

CLINICAL ALERT

   d. Aseptic technique is an added precaution to prevent contamination of a person, object, or site by microorganisms; it may include hand washing and the use of sterile gloves and dressing supplies for an open wound
8. Prevent transmission of infection by following CDC guidelines for infection control and isolation
9. Be aware that active immunization against hepatitis B is recommended for health care personnel who have intimate contact with people already infected and whose risk of infection with hepatitis B is substantial
10. Separate patients with a diagnosed infection, if possible, from other patients in the critical care unit to prevent cross-contamination
11. Provide patient teaching (for specific tips, see *Infection control*)

POINTS TO REMEMBER

- ♦ Intravascular catheter-related sepsis is the primary cause of septicemia in the critically ill patient.
- ♦ Approximately 50% of patients who become septic die as a result.
- ♦ Proper hand washing is the primary means to prevent infection transmission.

- Gloves are indicated to prevent skin and mucous membrane exposure to blood and body fluids.
- Patients should be strongly encouraged to inform others of a history of infection if it will have a major effect on health or lifestyle practices.

Study Questions

To evaluate your understanding of this chapter, answer the following questions in the space provided; then compare your responses with the correct answers in Appendix B, page 280.

1. What is the most common cause of septicemia in critically ill patients? ____
____
____

2. What information is provided by culture and sensitivity studies? ________
____
____

3. What is the primary means of preventing infection transmission? ________
____
____

Critical Thinking and Application Exercises

1. Consult with an infection-control nurse practitioner to identify institutional guidelines in the clinical setting.
2. Collect a specimen for culture and sensitivity studies according to your facility's collection protocol.
3. Prepare drug cards for the major antibiotic classifications.
4. Set up a sterile field for a dressing change; include the use of sterile gloves.

CHAPTER

6

Emergency Life Support: Resuscitation

Learning objectives

After studying this chapter, you should be able to:

- Describe the general principles related to the patient requiring resuscitation.
- Identify the common causes of cardiopulmonary arrest.
- Discuss the common physical assessment and diagnostic test findings used to determine the need for resuscitation.
- Describe care management for the patient requiring resuscitation.

Chapter overview

Cardiopulmonary resuscitation is indicated for cardiac arrest precipitated by any event. The American Heart Association defines Basic Cardiac Life Support (BCLS) as rescue breathing, obstructive airway maneuver, and chest compressions. Advanced Life Support is defined as BCLS plus adjunctive therapies to support circulation and ventilation; these therapies may include administration of I.V. fluids and drugs, defibrillation and cardiac monitoring, and intubation for airway support.

♦ I. Introduction

A. Cardiopulmonary resuscitation (CPR)
   1. CPR is indicated for cardiac arrest
   2. Cardiac arrest occurs when the heart stops beating (asystole) or when contractions are inadequate to maintain cardiac output, as in ventricular tachycardia or fibrillation
   3. Cardiac arrest may be precipitated by myocardial infarction (most common), heart failure, shock, severe electrolyte imbalance, acid-base imbalance, drowning, electrocution, drug overdose, or respiratory arrest
   4. Cardiac arrest is always immediately accompanied by respiratory arrest
   5. Respiratory arrest may be precipitated by airway obstruction, acute exacerbation of chronic airway disease, status asthmaticus, or drug overdose
   6. Respiratory arrest, if untreated, will precipitate cardiac arrest

B. Basic cardiac life support (BCLS)
   1. BCLS is emergency first aid that focuses on identifying respiratory or cardiac arrest and providing CPR until the victim responds or the next type of life support is initiated
   2. Life support, or CPR, follows an A-B-C sequence
      a. A — open the *airway* by lifting the jaw and tilting the head back (unless a neck injury is present)
      b. B — restore *breathing* by artificial ventilation (mouth-to-mouth resuscitation or a ventilatory assist device)
      c. C — restore *circulation* by delivering closed chest compressions
   3. All health professionals should be competent in BCLS skills

C. Advanced cardiac life support (ACLS)
   1. ACLS includes BCLS plus the use of adjunctive therapies to support ventilation, such as establishment of I.V. access, drug administration, cardiac monitoring, DEFIBRILLATION, control of arrhythmias, and postresuscitation care
   2. Specific procedures and therapeutic interventions and options for BCLS and ACLS are classified by the American Heart Association's Standards and Guidelines for Cardiopulmonary Resuscitation and Emergency Cardiac Care
      a. Class I: usually indicated, always acceptable, considered useful and effective
      b. Class II: acceptable, of uncertain efficiency, may be controversial; further divided into subclasses
         (1) IIa: evidence in favor of usefulness and efficacy, probably helpful

(2) IIb: not well established; may be helpful, probably not harmful

c. Class III: inappropriate, without supporting data, may be harmful

3. All doctors and nurses practicing in critical care and emergency areas must be competent in ACLS skills

CLINICAL ALERT

4. Optimal responses are achieved if BCLS is initiated within 4 minutes of the cardiac arrest, followed by ACLS within 8 minutes of the arrest

♦ II. Assessing the need for life support

A. Physical assessment findings

1. Unresponsiveness
2. Gasping or absent respiration
3. Lack of palpable carotid pulse and audible or palpable blood pressure

CLINICAL ALERT

   a. A pulse check must take at least 5 seconds
   b. A patient with bradycardia may have a slow and faint pulse that could be missed with a rapid pulse check
4. Arrhythmia (may include ventricular tachycardia or fibrillation, asystole, or pulseless electrical activity)

B. Diagnostic test findings

1. Arterial blood gas analysis: respiratory acidosis and hypoxemia
2. Electrocardiogram (ECG): ventricular tachycardia or fibrillation, asystole
3. Serum potassium levels: below or above normal; may precipitate arrhythmias
4. Serum calcium levels: low in patients on calcium channel blockers

♦ III. Patient care management

A. Goals

1. Restore effective breathing
2. Restore cardiac output

B. Possible nursing diagnoses

1. Decreased cardiac output
2. Altered tissue perfusion
3. Ineffective breathing pattern

C. Strategies

1. Initiate BCLS and ACLS according to American Heart Association guidelines
   a. Cardiac monitoring to identify arrhythmias
   b. Defibrillation by trained personnel on identification of arrhythmia or analysis or advisory of automatic defibrillation

TEACHING TIPS

After resuscitation

Be sure to include the following topics when preparing your teaching plan for the patient who has been resuscitated.

- Risk factors for and causes of cardiopulmonary arrest
- Fears and anxiety from a near-death experience
- BCLS training for family members
- Family preparation for seeing the patient after the event, including his physical appearance and inability to speak while intubated
- Equipment necessary to monitor and care for the patient
- Assistance of chaplain or clergy to be with the family

c. Intubation and oxygen administration to support ventilation

d. I.V. lifeline access (peripheral or central site) for administration of drugs and fluids

e. Drug therapy to treat cardiac arrhythmias, decreased cardiac output, and acid-base imbalances (for more details, see Appendix C, Identifying and Treating Arrhythmias, pages 289 to 291)

CLINICAL ALERT

f. Documentation of the therapy sequence and responses to therapy, according to institutional policy

2. Follow institutional policies that determine responsibilities in ACLS protocols
3. Support the family and help them prepare to see the patient by describing changes in appearance and the presence and purpose of endotracheal, nasogastric, or I.V. tubes
4. Provide patient teaching (for specific tips, see *After resuscitation*)

Points to remember

- ♦ Life support, or CPR, follows an A-B-C sequence: Airway, Breathing, and Circulation.
- ♦ Optimal responses from resuscitation are achieved if BCLS is initiated within 4 minutes of the cardiac arrest, followed by ACLS within 8 minutes of the cardiac arrest.
- ♦ The most common cause of sudden cardiac arrest is myocardial infarction.
- ♦ Family members of high-risk patients should learn to initiate BCLS.

STUDY QUESTIONS

To evaluate your understanding of this chapter, answer the following questions in the space provided; then compare your responses with the correct answers in Appendix B, page 280.

1. What is the sequence of CPR? ________________________________

2. What are the two types of emergency life support? ________________________________

3. Which assessment findings indicate a need for CPR? ________________________________

4. What information should nurses document for patients receiving BCLS or ACLS? ________________________________

CRITICAL THINKING AND APPLICATION EXERCISES

1. Complete a BCLS course.
2. Consult an ACLS manual to identify examples of each classification of ACLS procedures and therapeutic interventions.
3. Obtain a copy of a form for documenting resuscitation.
4. Interview a patient who has had a successful resuscitation. Prepare an oral class presentation describing the patient's and family's needs and how they were addressed.

CHAPTER

7

Mechanical Ventilation

Learning objectives

After studying this chapter, you should be able to:

- Explain the general principles that underlie mechanical ventilation.
- Identify different types of mechanical ventilators.
- Describe how common types of ventilators operate to support or control breathing.
- Describe diagnostic test findings used to assess the need for mechanical ventilation and monitor patients on mechanical ventilation.
- Discuss how to wean a patient from mechanical ventilation.
- Describe care management for the patient requiring mechanical ventilation.

Chapter overview

Mechanical ventilation artificially controls or supports breathing. Ventilators work by creating pressure changes that cause air to move into and out of the lungs. Specific diagnostic criteria help to identify patients who require mechanical ventilation. A variety of ventilator types, ventilation modes, and ventilatory adjuncts are available to meet the patient's individual needs for ventilatory support. Positive pressure, volume-cycled ventilators, the most commonly used type in adult patients, deliver a specific volume of air with each cycled ventilation. Weaning techniques focus on gradually increasing the patient's use of respiratory muscles and making sure that he can breathe without assistance before terminating mechanical ventilation.

♦ I. Introduction

A. Definition
   1. When a patient cannot provide adequate gas exchange to supply body tissues with oxygen, mechanical ventilation artificially supports or assists breathing
      a. Takes over the physical work of moving air into and out of the lungs
      b. Does not replace or alter physiologic lung function
   2. A doctor selects a ventilator type and mode based on the patient's diagnosis and specific needs
   3. The ventilator is connected to an artificial airway
      a. An oral or a nasal endotracheal (ET) tube is used for short-term ventilation (cuffed for adults; uncuffed for children)
      b. A tracheostomy tube is used for long-term ventilation

B. Purpose
   1. To provide mechanical power that will enable the pulmonary system to maintain ventilation when a neurologic or neuromuscular condition or pharmacologically induced paralysis prevents breathing
   2. To improve the efficiency of ventilation or oxygenation by manipulating the ventilatory pattern and airway pressures
   3. To provide hyperventilation for a patient with head injuries

C. Complications
   1. PNEUMOTHORAX may result from alveolar rupture caused by high positive pressure required to deliver a preset volume
   2. Barotrauma may result from increased intrathoracic pressure, which can damage major vessels or organs in the thorax
   3. Alterations in hemodynamic pressure may result from increased intrathoracic pressure, which can impede venous return, thereby leading to decreased cardiac output and increased pulmonary artery wedge pressure
   4. Increased intracranial pressure may result from decreased venous return and blood pooling in the cerebral vessels
   5. Water imbalance may result from humidified air use, reduced lymphatic flow, or syndrome of inappropriate antidiuretic hormone

♦ II. Types and modes of ventilation

A. Types of ventilators
   1. Negative pressure: exerts negative pressure on the external chest (iron lung or cuirass); does not require intubation; rarely used today
   2. Positive pressure, pressure-cycled: exerts positive pressure on the airway; a predetermined pressure terminates inspiration and may prohibit delivery of TIDAL VOLUME
   3. Positive pressure, time-cycled: exerts positive pressure on the airway; delivers a volume of gas over a predetermined time
   4. Positive pressure, volume-cycled: exerts positive pressure on the airway; delivers a predetermined volume of gas and allows limits to be set for pressure and time; the most commonly used type of ventilator
   5. Positive pressure, jet ventilation: exerts positive pressure on the airway; delivers small volumes of gas at very high rates

B. Modes of ventilation
   1. *Controlled mandatory ventilation (CMV)*: delivers a preset tidal volume at a preset rate; ignores the patient's own ventilatory effort; least frequently used mode of ventilation
   2. *Assist controlled ventilation (ACV)*: delivers a preset tidal volume for every breath initiated by the machine or through the patient's effort; allows hyperventilation
   3. *Intermittent mandatory ventilation (IMV)*: delivers a preset tidal volume at a preset rate while allowing the patient to breathe at his own rate and tidal volume; breath stacking may occur if ventilation is out of sync with the patient's own efforts
   4. *Synchronized intermittent mandatory ventilation (SIMV)*: delivers a preset, mandatory tidal volume synchronized to the patient's inspiratory effort; the most commonly used mode of ventilation

C. Ventilatory adjuncts
   1. Positive end-expiratory pressure (PEEP): positive pressure exerted by mechanical ventilation at the end of expiration; counteracts small airway collapse and facilitates gas exchange to improve oxygenation
   2. Continuous positive airway pressure (CPAP): positive pressure exerted continuously by mechanical ventilation; helps prevent alveolar collapse in spontaneously breathing patients
   3. Pressure support: positive pressure exerted by mechanical ventilation at the beginning of inspiration; used to minimize stress caused by breathing through an artificial airway

D. Ventilator controls

1. Mode: selection of CMV, ACV, IMV, or SIMV
2. F_{IO_2}: the fraction of inspired oxygen; usually reported as a percentage (.40 = 40%)
3. Tidal volume: the amount of air delivered to the patient with each inspiratory cycle; the amount of tidal volume set on a ventilator is 10 to 15 ml/kg of body weight
4. Rate: the number of ventilator breaths delivered each minute; the patient's spontaneous rate is added to the ventilator rate to obtain the actual respiratory rate per minute
5. Peak inspiratory pressure: the amount of pressure exerted to deliver a preset tidal volume; limits are set to prevent barotrauma; remaining volume will not be delivered when pressure limit is reached
6. Alarms: the safety devices used to monitor alterations in rate, volume, and pressure; these vary from machine to machine
7. Inspiratory/expiratory (I:E) ratio: compares the duration of inspiration with the duration of expiration; normal ratio is 1:2; note that expiration is twice as long as inspiration

♦ III. Assessing the need for mechanical ventilation

A. Physical assessment findings

1. Dyspnea
2. Tachypnea
3. Adventitious or absent breath sounds
4. Cyanosis
5. Alteration in mental status
6. Tachycardia or other arrhythmia secondary to hypoxia

B. Diagnostic test findings

1. Arterial blood gas (ABG) levels: partial pressure of carbon dioxide (Pa_{CO_2}) greater than 50; partial pressure of oxygen (Pa_{O_2}) less than 50; pH less than 7.35

CLINICAL ALERT

   a. Arterial oxygen saturation (Sa_{O_2}) less than 80
   b. Decreased level of consciousness, increased respiratory rate, and decreased Sa_{O_2} provide early indication of respiratory distress

2. Tidal volume: less than 5 ml/kg
3. Negative inspiratory force (NIF): less than 20 cm H_2O
4. Minute volume (tidal volume × rate): less than 10 liters/minute

♦ IV. Weaning the patient from mechanical ventilation

A. IMV

1. The ventilatory rate is decreased gradually as the patient becomes able to resume the work of breathing
2. Usually best for the patient on long-term ventilatory support

B. T-piece adapter placed on an ET tube with supplemental oxygen
1. The patient is taken off the ventilator and must breathe spontaneously for increasing periods; afterward, the patient is returned to the ventilator to permit rest
2. Usually used for postoperative patients who undergo mechanical ventilation for a short time until anesthetic effects wear off or for patients who undergo pharmacologic paralysis during a short procedure

♦ V. Patient care management

A. Goals of mechanical ventilation
1. Decrease the work of breathing
2. Improve gas exchange and tissue perfusion

B. Suggested nursing diagnoses for a patient requiring mechanical ventilation
1. Ineffective airway clearance
2. Anxiety
3. Ineffective breathing pattern
4. Impaired gas exchange
5. Risk for infection
6. Impaired verbal communication
7. Activity intolerance

C. Strategies
1. Verify and maintain the ventilator settings according to the doctor's order and institutional policy
   a. Mode
   b. FIO_2
   c. Tidal volume
   d. Rate
   e. Ventilatory adjuncts, such as PEEP and CPAP
   f. Alarms
2. Monitor SaO_2 with pulse oximeter
   a. Sensor attaches to nose, temple, or finger
   b. Alarm parameters may be determined for heart rate and saturation
   c. Continuously monitors heart rate and oxygen saturation and displays findings (normal SaO_2 is 95% to 100%)
3. Suction as necessary to remove secretions
   a. Assess and auscultate for presence of fluid, mucus, or obstruction before suctioning (to determine if necessary) and after (to assess effectiveness of suctioning)
   b. Hyperoxygenate and ventilate before suctioning to prevent hypoxia

   c. Observe the patient carefully for decreases in heart rate and SaO_2 during suctioning
   d. In-line suction devices decrease the risk for infection and may decrease the potential for hypoxia
4. Assess the following and document findings: continuous electrocardiogram (ECG) rhythm; vital signs; mental status; heart, lung, and bowel sounds; urine output; patient's comfort level
5. If a pulmonary artery catheter is in place, assess and document hemodynamic status and pressures
6. Administer drug therapy, as prescribed
   a. Bronchodilators to dilate smooth muscle of large airways
   b. Neuromuscular blocking agents, such as vecuronium bromide (Norcuron) and atracurium besylate (Tracrium), to further decrease the work of breathing and maximize the use of mechanical ventilation
   c. Diuretics to reduce circulating fluid and volume overload
   d. Antibiotics to fight infection, if necessary
   e. Analgesics to alleviate pain after an operative procedure or from another cause; administer nonnarcotic analgesics when possible

CLINICAL ALERT

7. As prescribed, administer sedatives to patients who receive neuromuscular blocking agents to decrease anxiety about being paralyzed and unable to move
8. Insert a nasogastric tube to relieve gastric distention and prevent aspiration
9. Administer enteral or parenteral nutrition to support the patient's metabolic needs and fight infection
   a. Administer enteral nutrition by feeding tube if the patient's GI tract is functioning
   b. Administer parenteral nutrition by a central venous or peripheral line if the patient's GI tract is not functioning
10. To determine the adequacy of ventilation, monitor ABG levels for indications of hypoxia and acid-base imbalance
11. Place the patient in low Fowler's or semi-Fowler's position to improve comfort and to facilitate respiration
12. Troubleshoot *high-pressure ventilator alarms*, which may indicate the following:
   a. Patient requires suctioning
   b. Tubing is kinked
   c. Water or secretions are in tubing
   d. Patient is biting ET tube
   e. Patient has bronchospasm or cough
   f. Patient has decreased lung compliance requiring higher inspiratory pressures

(Text continues on page 54.)

DECISION TREE

Troubleshooting high-pressure ventilator alarms

Alarms are used to monitor changes in rate, rhythm, and pressure and to help ensure ventilator safety. Types of alarms vary from one machine to another. If an alarm sounds, assess the situation and take appropriate nursing actions immediately. The decision tree below shows the troubleshooting process for a high-pressure ventilator alarm.

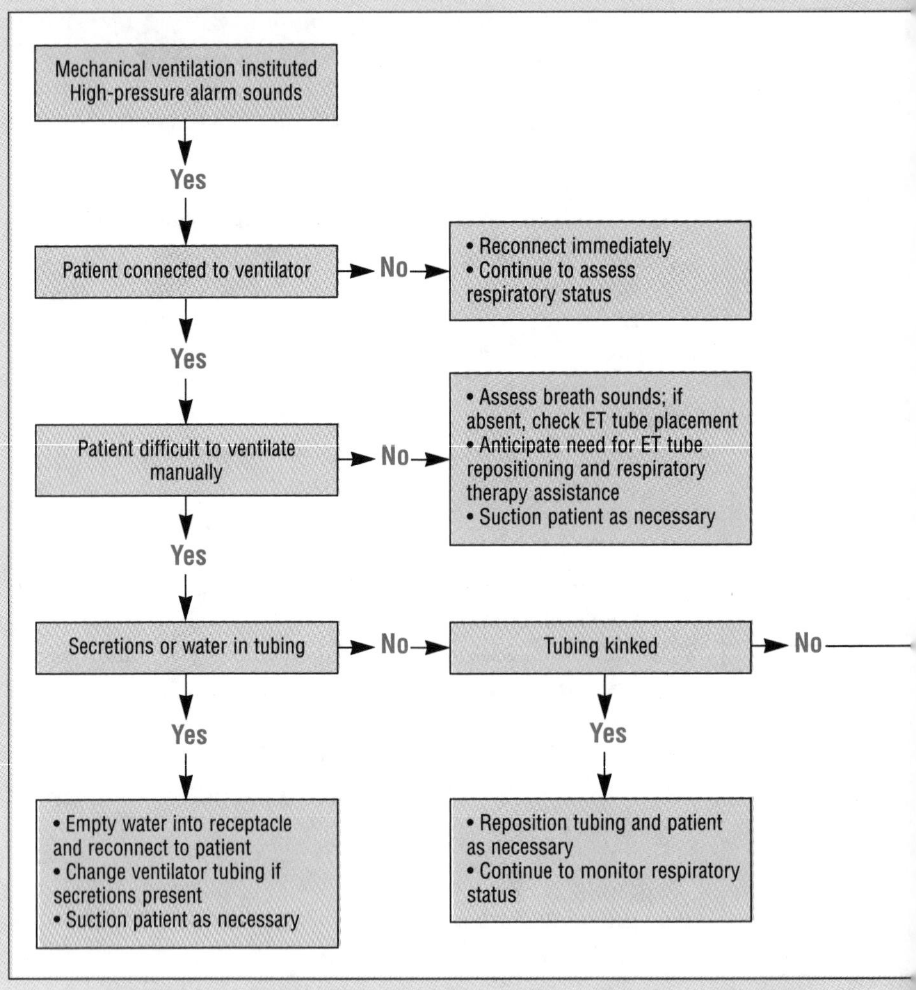

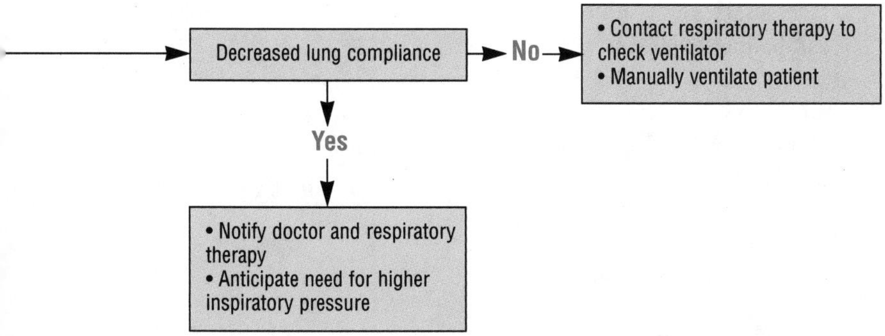
Decreased lung compliance
No
• Contact respiratory therapy to check ventilator
• Manually ventilate patient
Yes
• Notify doctor and respiratory therapy
• Anticipate need for higher inspiratory pressure

TEACHING TIPS

Patient undergoing mechanical ventilation

Be sure to include the following topics when preparing your teaching plan for the patient undergoing mechanical ventilation.

- Muscle retraining and relaxation techniques to support breathing
- Importance of remaining calm and allowing the ventilator to assist and support ventilation
- Communication methods
- Reason for frequent assessments of level of consciousness and specimens for laboratory analysis
- Possible need for long-term ventilatory support
- Pain control and the need to use agents with minimal respiratory depressive effects
- Adequate rest and nutrition
- How to perform breathing techniques

13. Troubleshoot *low-pressure ventilator alarms,* which may indicate the following:
    a. Tubing is disconnected from machine circuit or from patient
    b. ET tube cuff has a leak

CLINICAL ALERT

14. Be aware that when a ventilator alarm sounds, the ventilator terminates delivery of the prescribed volume of gas; if the alarm sounds frequently, the patient may not be receiving the prescribed tidal volume/minute ventilation (for more information, see *Troubleshooting high-pressure ventilator alarms,* pages 52 and 53)
15. If necessary, apply soft restraints to protect the patient from self-extubation; follow institutional policy
16. Offer the intubated patient frequent mouth care and comfort measures
17. Communicate using simple yes-or-no questions, gestures, and a word or letter board
18. Assess readiness to wean
    a. NIF: greater than -20 cm H_2O
    b. Tidal volume: greater than 15 ml/kg
    c. FIO_2: less than 40%
    d. ABG levels: $PaCO_2$ of 45 mm Hg or less, PaO_2 of 60 mm Hg or greater, and pH of 7.35 to 7.45 (ABG levels for patients with chronic obstructive pulmonary disease may not be within normal parameters; ABG levels should be near patient's baseline)
19. Provide emotional support to decrease the patient's fear and anxiety
20. Provide patient teaching (for specific tips, see *Patient undergoing mechanical ventilation*)

Points to remember

- Mechanical ventilation takes over the physical work of breathing but does not alter physiologic lung function.
- Positive-pressure, volume-cycled ventilators are the most commonly used ventilators for adults.
- SIMV is the most commonly used mode of mechanical ventilation.
- Pneumothorax is a common complication of mechanical ventilation.
- Hyperoxygenation and hyperventilation before suctioning decrease the risk for hypoxia.

Study questions

To evaluate your understanding of this chapter, answer the following questions in the space provided; then compare your responses with the correct answers in Appendix B, page 281.

1. What are the hemodynamic complications of mechanical ventilation? ____

___

___

2. Which type of mechanical ventilator is most commonly used? ____

___

___

3. Which mode of mechanical ventilation is most commonly used? ____

___

___

4. What diagnostic test findings indicate the need for mechanical ventilation?

___

___

5. When should a patient on a mechanical ventilator be suctioned? ____

___

___

6. What are the indicators of a patient's readiness to be weaned from a mechanical ventilator? ______________________________

____

____

CRITICAL THINKING AND APPLICATION EXERCISES

1. Determine the types of ventilator and modes of ventilation most commonly used in your institution. Consider interviewing respiratory therapy or ventilator support staff.
2. Observe a patient being suctioned for changes in vital signs and SaO_2.
3. Perform the procedure for suctioning a patient who is mechanically ventilated using an in-line suction system, if available, and a traditional suction catheter.
4. Identify the following parameters (ventilator settings) for a patient: mode, rate, FIO_2, tidal volume, PEEP/CPAP, and pressure support. Obtain the information from the ventilator itself (not from the doctor's order).
5. Find out which devices for securing ET tubes are available in the clinical setting.

CHAPTER

8

Hemodynamic Monitoring

Learning objectives

After studying this chapter, you should be able to:

- Identify the basic principles of hemodynamic monitoring.
- List the information obtained through hemodynamic monitoring.
- Discuss the primary uses for each type of hemodynamic monitoring.
- Discuss the implications of readings obtained for each type of hemodynamic monitoring.
- Describe patient care management for each type of hemodynamic monitoring.

Chapter overview

Hemodynamic monitoring is an invasive technique for measuring pressures and values within the heart, lungs, and circulatory system. Pressure readings obtained during hemodynamic monitoring are compared with the patient's baseline values as well as normal values. Performed in critical care units and emergency departments, hemodynamic monitoring is a specialized nursing skill.

♦ I. Introduction

A. Physiologic concepts
1. Each chamber of the heart and the arterial system have normal pressures; these pressures are measured by hemodynamic monitoring
2. During hemodynamic monitoring, a fluid-filled catheter is inserted into an artery or one of the heart's chambers; the fluid-filled catheter transmits pressure readings to a TRANSDUCER, which converts the pressure readings into an electrical signal represented by waveforms on a bedside monitor
3. A doctor or nurse reads hemodynamic waveforms on the bedside monitor and compares findings with normal values and with the patient's baseline values
4. Information obtained from hemodynamic monitoring helps to evaluate the function and performance of the heart and the circulatory system

CLINICAL ALERT

5. Trends in readings correlated to the patient's clinical condition provide more useful information than isolated readings

B. Uses
1. To monitor directly cardiovascular pressures
2. To guide nursing interventions, such as assessment of fluid status and the titration of drugs
3. To assess treatment effectiveness by evaluating trends in obtained values
4. To monitor the patient's progress by evaluating pressure waveforms and values

C. General patient care management
1. Obtain INFORMED CONSENT for hemodynamic monitoring
2. Assess the patient's understanding of the rationale for catheter insertion; use this information to prepare a teaching plan
3. To prepare for insertion, set up the equipment according to institutional policy; aseptic technique is essential for line insertion and maintenance
4. Observe the patient for anxiety and evidence of complications
5. Assess the results of therapeutic interventions, and make changes to fluids, drug therapy, or treatment measures, as ordered
6. Record pressure data and vital signs according to the patient's condition and institutional policy

CLINICAL ALERT

7. Level, zero, and CALIBRATE the equipment to ensure accurate data at least once a shift or when values are questionable; level the transducer to the PHLEBOSTATIC AXIS, known as the ZERO REFERENCE POINT
8. Maintain a fluid-filled pressure system to ensure accurate transmission of the pressure signal because air in the pressure system that is allowed to enter the patient will create an air embolus

TEACHING TIPS

Patient undergoing hemodynamic monitoring

Be sure to include both the patient and family members as part of your teaching. Acknowledge their fears, and answer all questions honestly. Your teaching should cover the following topics.

- Rationale for hemodynamic monitoring and associated nursing activities
- Need for frequent monitoring of the patient's status and the effects of therapy
- Alarms and what they mean
- Signs and symptoms to report to the nurse

9. Change pressure system fluids, tubing, and dressings according to institutional policy
10. Assess the patient and waveforms frequently for changes from the baseline assessment to prevent complications; these changes are regarded as trends
11. Notify the doctor when parameters are outside acceptable ranges
12. Provide patient teaching (see *Patient undergoing hemodynamic monitoring*)

♦ II. Arterial pressure monitoring

A. General information

1. Arterial pressure may be measured indirectly with a blood pressure cuff and stethoscope or an automatic blood pressure–measuring device
2. Direct intra-arterial measurement may be taken after inserting a cannula into an artery and connecting the cannula to a pressure-monitoring device (intra-arterial monitoring is discussed in this section)
3. The catheter is inserted through the radial, brachial, or femoral artery
4. The radial artery is the preferred insertion site because that artery is small and superficial, with good collateral circulation
5. The brachial artery is a less desirable insertion site because that artery is deeper and more difficult to cannulate
6. The femoral artery is the least desirable insertion site because that artery is the largest and deepest of the three; is close to the femoral vein; and has no collateral circulation, so blood flow to the body area it supplies is compromised if complications occur
7. Regulation of arterial pressure involves neurohormonal control, which affects the volume of blood flow through the vessels and the elasticity of the resistance vessels

8. Systolic blood pressure (SBP) is the highest pressure occurring within the arterial system during a cardiac cycle; SBP determines the perfusion pressure on body tissues; SBP is an indirect indicator of stroke volume
9. Diastolic blood pressure (DBP) is the lowest pressure occurring within the arterial system during a cardiac cycle; DBP is an indirect indicator of systemic vascular resistance
10. The right coronary, left anterior descending, and circumflex arteries perfuse throughout the cardiac cycle; subendocardial vessels, however, only perfuse during diastole, often leading to subendocardial ischemia
11. Pulse pressure is the difference between SBP and DBP (normally 40 to 60 mm Hg) and reflects the vascular resistance of the arterial system and the stroke volume
12. Mean arterial pressure (MAP) is the average pressure under which blood flows to the tissue during the cardiac cycle; it is calculated by the formula

$$MAP = \frac{SBP + 2DBP}{3}$$

CLINICAL ALERT

13. A MAP of at least 60 mm Hg is necessary to maintain autoregulation in the heart, brain, and kidneys

B. Uses
1. Monitors direct intra-arterial pressures
2. Provides more accurate information about vascular capacity, blood volume, and heart pumping effectiveness
3. Allows routine blood specimens to be obtained from the line, which prevents the need for repeated needlesticks

C. Normal waveforms
1. A normal arterial waveform, noted by intra-arterial monitoring, consists of a rapid, sharp upstroke, a dicrotic notch (DN), and a clear end-diastole; heart rate and rhythm may alter waveform configuration
2. The baseline of the wave is the aortic end-diastolic pressure (AEDP), indicating the minimum pressure reached in the arteries during diastole
3. The top of the wave is the peak systolic pressure (PSP), indicating the maximum pressure reached in the arteries during systole; PSP is heard as SBP
4. The DN signifies the beginning of diastole (see *Normal arterial waveform*)

Normal arterial waveform

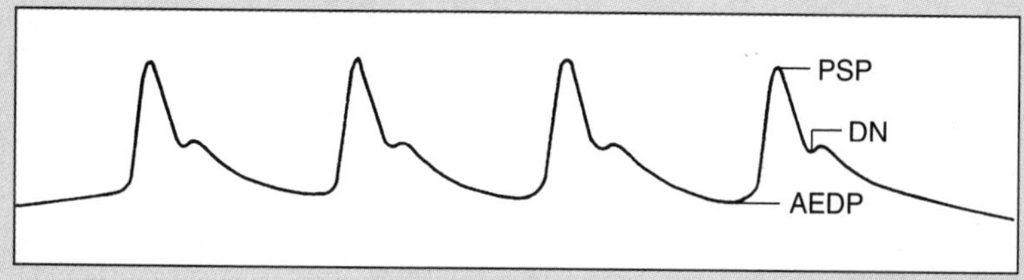

D. Implications of abnormal waveforms and readings

1. For a patient in shock, SBP by cuff measurement is less accurate than intra-arterial SBP; the difference may be greater in a patient with increased systemic vascular resistance caused by alpha-adrenergic stimulation, which may occur in a patient receiving vasopressors to increase blood pressure
2. Intra-arterial SBP of less than 80 mm Hg, or 30 mm Hg less than the patient's normal SBP, indicates shock
3. Intra-arterial SBP of greater than 150 mm Hg or a DBP greater than 100 mm Hg signifies hypertension

E. Patient care management

1. Do not insert any medications (except heparin flush solution) through the intra-arterial line
2. Level the air-fluid interface of the transducer at the catheter tip before obtaining readings for peripheral blood pressures; level the interface at the phlebostatic axis before obtaining readings for aortic root or central blood pressure
3. Remove all air from the tubing and transducer because air bubbles dampen or distort the waveform
4. Depending on institutional policy, you may use a heparinized low-flow flush solution (1 to 2 units/ml) to maintain line patency and normal waveform transmission
5. Calibrate the transducer to a known pressure to ensure accurate pressure readings; compare arterial line pressures with sphygmomanometer pressures at least once per shift; use correctly functioning intra-arterial line pressures, when possible, because they are more accurate than cuff pressures

CLINICAL ALERT

6. Keep in mind that a dampened waveform (indicated by loss of the DN or a flattened upstroke) indicates air, blood, or clots in the arterial line
7. Stabilize the catheter position with a dressing to prevent kinking and to increase accuracy of reading
8. Use luer-lock connectors to prevent breaks in the monitoring setup

9. Obtain routine blood specimens from the line
10. Monitor for possible complications, such as infection, hemorrhage, decreased or absent pulses distal to the insertion site, embolus, and thrombus
11. Check collateral circulation by performing Allen's test before inserting a catheter into the radial artery
12. Keep in mind that brachial or femoral artery cannulation requires immobilization of the patient's affected arm, limiting range of motion and self-care activities
13. Remember that bleeding from femoral artery cannulation may be more difficult to control because of the difficulty in applying adequate pressure to the site, that large amounts of blood can be lost in the thigh before external signs of bleeding are evident, and that the site's proximity to the perineal area exposes it to bacterial contamination

♦ III. Central venous pressure (CVP) monitoring

A. General information
1. CVP is measured by a manometer connected to a central line or by a transducer connected to the proximal lumen of a pulmonary artery catheter; the catheter is located in the superior vena cava or the right atrium
2. CVP is measured in millimeters of mercury (mm Hg) or centimeters of water (cm H_2O); to convert from one to the other, use this equivalence: 1 mm Hg equals 1.36 cm H_2O
3. Using a water manometer to assess CVP (most common method) involves measuring the height of a column of water in a plastic or glass manometer with a three-way stopcock connected to a central line and attached to the I.V. tubing
4. CVP represents the filling pressure or preload of the right ventricle or right ventricular end-diastolic pressure
5. CVP can be used to assess fluid volume status because the venous bed contains 60% of blood volume
6. CVP may be the last pressure to change in a patient with a rapidly changing cardiovascular status

CLINICAL ALERT

7. CVP is an unreliable indicator of left-sided heart pressures

B. Uses
1. Evaluates right atrial and right ventricular pressure and function
2. Monitors blood volume
3. Assesses adequacy of central venous return
4. Guides fluid volume administration by evaluating trends in the values obtained
5. May differentiate right ventricular failure from left ventricular failure

C. Normal readings: 4 to 10 cm H_2O; 3 to 7 mm Hg

D. Implications of abnormal readings
   1. CVP is an unreliable indicator of left ventricular function
   2. CVP lower than 4 cm H_2O may indicate hypovolemia
   3. CVP higher than 10 cm H_2O may indicate hypervolemia or poor myocardial contractility

E. Patient care management
   1. Level the zero mark on the manometer to the phlebostatic axis for accuracy
   2. Indicate the level of the phlebostatic axis with an ink mark on the chest to ensure consistent readings
   3. Do not allow the manometer to overflow because this may cause contamination
   4. Observe for fluctuation of the fluid level with respiration; the level will drop with inspiration and rise with expiration from intrathoracic pressure changes
   5. Record pressures at the end of expiration after the fluid level stops fluctuating
   6 Observe for signs of common complications, such as infection and air embolism

♦ IV. Pulmonary artery pressure (PAP) monitoring

A. General information
   1. PAP is measured by a pulmonary artery (PA) catheter
   2. A PA catheter has a balloon tip with two to seven lumens or ports
   3. The catheter is passed through a large vein, such as the internal jugular or subclavian vein, into the right atrium of the heart
   4. Once within the right atrium, the balloon is inflated and the catheter is advanced through the heart into the PA; when waveforms indicate that the tip of the catheter is in the PA, the catheter is secured; the balloon is deflated during continuous monitoring
   5. When readings are taken, the balloon is inflated and the catheter "floats" out to occlude a smaller branch of the PA, allowing for measurement of pressure in front of the balloon; this pressure is called the pulmonary artery wedge pressure (PAWP), also known as the pulmonary capillary wedge pressure or pulmonary artery occlusive pressure

B. Uses
   1. Monitors direct intracardiac pressures
   2. Provides information about vascular capacity, blood volume, pump effectiveness, and tissue perfusion
   3. Indirectly reflects left ventricular end-diastolic pressure (LVEDP), which indicates left ventricular function

Pulmonary artery catheter waveforms

RIGHT ATRIAL PRESSURE	RIGHT VENTRICULAR PRESSURE	PULMONARY ARTERY PRESSURE	PULMONARY ARTERY WEDGE PRESSURE
Normal Range			
Mean: 3 to 6 mm Hg Waveform seen when the catheter tip reaches the right atrium.	Systolic: 17 to 32 mm Hg Diastolic: 1 to 7 mm Hg Waveform seen when the balloon-inflated catheter tip reaches the right ventricle.	Systolic: 17 to 32 mm Hg Diastolic: 4 to 13 mm Hg Mean: 9 to 19 mm Hg Waveform seen when the balloon-inflated catheter tip reaches the pulmonary artery.	Mean: 8 to 12 mm Hg Waveform seen when the balloon wedges in a smaller branch of the pulmonary artery.

4. The distal tip of the catheter measures PAP and PAWP; mixed venous blood specimens can be obtained from this port
5. The proximal port is used for continuous infusion of fluids or medications; it measures right atrial pressure with a stopcock configuration when the distal tip is in the PA

C. Normal readings and waveforms: each pressure has a characteristic waveform
1. Mean right atrial pressure: 3 to 6 mm Hg
2. PAP: systolic, 17 to 32 mm Hg; diastolic, 4 to 13 mm Hg; mean, 9 to 19 mm Hg
3. PAWP: 8 to 12 mm Hg (see *Pulmonary artery catheter waveforms*)

PAWP 8-12

D. Implications of abnormal readings
1. In the absence of mitral disease, the mean PAWP closely approximates the LVEDP because the mitral valve is open during diastole and pressure in the left atrium is equal to pressure in the left ventricle
2. The LVEDP correlates with the ventricular volume; variations in the PAWP indicate the earliest changes in left ventricular filling and function
3. The PA diastolic pressure is normally 1 to 4 mm Hg higher than the PAWP; in the absence of lung disease, this pressure can be used to evaluate left ventricular function

CLINICAL ALERT

4. PAWP cannot be greater than PA diastolic pressure because of the pressure gradient within the heart and lungs

E. Patient care management

1. Read pressures at the end of expiration because intrathoracic pressure changes from breathing, mechanical ventilation, or positive end-expiratory pressure will alter PAP and PAWP
2. Keep in mind that right ventricular pressure readings (normal systolic is 17 to 32 mm Hg; normal diastolic is 1 to 7 mm Hg) are obtained only during catheter insertion
3. Level the air-fluid interface of the transducer at the phlebostatic axis before obtaining readings because an inverse change of 3 to 5 mm Hg is obtained for every inch of deviation from the established axis
4. Remove all air from the tubing and transducer while setting up and monitoring because air bubbles dampen or distort the waveform
5. Depending on institutional policy, you may use a heparinized low-flow flush solution (1 to 2 units/ml) to maintain line patency and normal waveform transmission
6. Calibrate the transducer to a known pressure to ensure accurate pressure readings
7. Stabilize the catheter position with a dressing to prevent kinking, to increase accuracy of the readings, and to minimize accidental dose fluctuations
8. Inflate the balloon slowly while observing waveforms only to the point that occlusion (wedge) is obtained (do not exceed maximum balloon volume); this prevents overwedging and, possibly, pulmonary infarction
9. Do not aspirate the air from an inflated balloon; remove the syringe and allow the balloon to deflate passively to avoid balloon rupture
10. Keep the balloon inflated no longer than necessary (less than 15 seconds) to prevent overwedging and, possibly, pulmonary infarction
11. Read the PAP and PAWP directly from hard copy or from a calibrated oscilloscope; digital readouts are unreliable and do not reflect the end of expiration (pressures are averaged and updated digitally every 4 seconds)
12. Avoid obtaining routine blood specimens from the catheter to decrease the risk of clotting and to ensure line patency

CLINICAL ALERT

13. Recognize that the patient is electrically sensitive with the catheter in place; a catheter entering the heart increases the risk of microshock, possibly producing ventricular fibrillation
14. Monitor for complications, such as arrhythmias, infection, air embolus, pneumothorax, and catheter clotting or kinking
15. Notify the doctor if displayed waveforms show a permanent PAWP reading, right ventricular pressure tracing, or PAWP outside the given parameters

♦ V. Cardiac output determination

A. General information

1. CARDIAC OUTPUT (CO) is the amount of blood the heart pumps per minute and is the product of the heart rate multiplied by stroke volume
2. Serial CO determinations provide valuable information about left ventricular function
3. The most common method used in a critical care area to measure CO is the thermodilution method, using the thermistor hub of the PA catheter
4. Thermodilution is based on this principle: If a known amount of solution at a known temperature is injected into the bloodstream, the speed at which the solution moves can be reported as a temperature change downstream; a CO computer connected to the thermistor hub port of the PA catheter calculates the speed of this temperature change
5. Iced injectate or room-temperature injectate can be used; a computation constant set on the CO computer can be changed to accommodate variations in temperature, volume, and catheter size
6. Advantages include rapid, reliable results unaffected by oxygen; no need to withdraw blood; only one person is needed to perform the procedure
7. Disadvantages include inaccuracy with low CO and with mitral or tricuspid insufficiency or shunts; procedure may pose an electrical hazard
8. Because CO varies among individuals, the cardiac index (CI) standardizes the CO results; patients with different body sizes can be compared. CI is calculated by dividing the CO by the body surface area (obtained from a standard chart) to adjust for body size

CLINICAL ALERT

9. CI is a more precise measurement than CO and is more commonly used to evaluate the patient's status

B. Uses

1. Assesses left ventricular function
2. Evaluates the adequacy of CO to help determine the extent of oxygen delivery to the tissues
3. Assesses the patient's response to therapy

C. Normal readings

1. CO: 4 to 8 liters/minute
2. CI: 2.5 to 4.0 liters/minute/m^2

D. Implications of abnormal readings
1. CI less than 2.2 liters/minute/m^2 indicates hypoperfusion to the tissues
2. CI less than 1.8 liters/minute/m^2 suggests cardiogenic shock
3. CI greater than 4.3 liters/minute/m^2 may be found in the early stages of septic shock or in situations in which the heart is compensating for increased metabolic demands (thyrotoxicosis, fever, exercise, and certain tumors)

E. Patient care management
1. Measure the volume of injectate exactly to ensure accurate results
2. Ensure that the computation constant is set at the correct number for volume and temperature of injectate
3. Monitor the injectate's temperature carefully so that the computer can correctly calculate any temperature change
4. Ensure representative CO measurements by taking three measurements and averaging the results; measurements should be within 10% of one another; any readings outside this range should not be counted
5. Inject the solution at end-expiration to negate the effects of intrathoracic pressure
6. Cover the electrical port of the PA catheter with the cap when the computer cable is disconnected to reduce the risk of microshock

♦ VI. Mixed venous oxygen saturation ($S\bar{v}O_2$) measurements

A. General information
1. Continuous mixed $S\bar{v}O_2$ assesses the balance between oxygen supply and tissue demand for oxygen; it reflects the body's ability to meet tissue oxygen needs
2. A fiberoptic PA catheter is used to measure the average percentage of oxygen bound to hemoglobin in venous blood
3. Its measurement indicates overall tissue oxygen and is recorded by an oximeter
4. An oximeter produces a digital readout of $S\bar{v}O_2$, along with a strip recorder, to provide a permanent written record
5. $S\bar{v}O_2$ is influenced by two primary factors: oxygen transport and tissue oxygen consumption
6. A change in one or both of these factors triggers compensation, producing changes in the $S\bar{v}O_2$ level

B. Uses
1. Aids in diagnosis and treatment of a critical care patient with a life-threatening condition, such as shock
2. Can serve as an early guide to intervention because changes in $S\bar{v}O_2$ values reflect changes in oxygen demand or delivery

3. May reduce repetitive arterial blood sampling, which can contribute to significant blood loss and cost

C. Normal readings: normal mixed $S\bar{v}O_2$ level is 60% to 80%

D. Implications of abnormal readings

1. Changes in venous oxygen pressure — even in small amounts — produce large changes in $S\bar{v}O_2$ levels
2. Decreased $S\bar{v}O_2$ levels reflect problems associated with increased oxygen demands or decreased oxygen delivery caused by a decrease in hemoglobin, arterial oxygen saturation, or CO
3. Decreased $S\bar{v}O_2$ levels can occur in a patient with anemia, hyperthermia, seizures, fever, shivering, arrhythmias, or heart failure
4. Increased $S\bar{v}O_2$ levels reflect problems associated with increased oxygen delivery, artifact, decreased oxygen uptake, and increased CO
5. Increased $S\bar{v}O_2$ levels can occur in a patient with polycythemia, anesthesia, hypothermia, left-to-right shunt, inotropic drug administration, increased fraction of inspired oxygen from mechanical ventilation, or septic shock

E. Patient care management

1. Evaluate the effects of nursing interventions (such as suctioning, personal care activities, changes in oxygen therapy delivery, and drug administration) on $S\bar{v}O_2$ readings
2. Complications related to $S\bar{v}O_2$ monitoring are associated with PAP monitoring (see "Patient care management," page 65, for other considerations)

POINTS TO REMEMBER

- Frequency of hemodynamic measurements is determined by the patient's clinical condition.
- Pressure values obtained should be assessed in relation to the patient's baseline hemodynamic pressure and should be viewed as trends.
- Actions based on data obtained by hemodynamic monitoring should be supported by other assessment findings.
- The clinical reliability of hemodynamic readings is directly related to the consistency and accuracy of the interpreter's measurements.

STUDY QUESTIONS

To evaluate your understanding of this chapter, answer the following questions in the space provided; then compare your responses with the correct answers in Appendix B, page 281.

1. What is the preferred insertion site for arterial pressure monitoring?

2. What are the components of a normal arterial waveform?

3. What does a CVP reading represent?

4. Why should the nurse allow the balloon of a PA catheter to deflate passively?

5. What do continuous mixed $S\bar{v}O_2$ measurements assess?

CRITICAL THINKING AND APPLICATION EXERCISES

1. Plot a patient's hemodynamic parameters for a 24-hour period, and relate the findings to the patient's clinical status.

2. Examine a PA catheter in the skills laboratory and identify the various ports and the thermistor head.

3. Develop a chart listing the patient care management for each type of hemodynamic monitoring.

4. Observe the effects of suctioning on mixed $S\bar{v}O_2$ measurements in a patient with a fiberoptic PA catheter.

CHAPTER

9

Intracranial Pressure Monitoring

Learning objectives

After studying this chapter, you should be able to:

- Identify the basic principles of intracranial pressure (ICP) monitoring.
- Describe advantages and disadvantages for each method of ICP monitoring.
- List the general information obtained through ICP monitoring.
- Describe care management for the patient being monitored for ICP.

Chapter overview

Effective management of patients undergoing intracranial pressure (ICP) monitoring requires a solid understanding of the physiology of the brain. Because the brain is enclosed in a cranial vault, changes in the volume of one of the components (brain tissue, cerebrospinal fluid, or blood volume) cause an increase in total pressure unless a reciprocal change occurs in another component. Different methods of ICP monitoring include intraventricular monitoring, subarachnoid screw monitoring, and epidural monitoring. Each method has advantages and disadvantages.

♦ I. Introduction

A. Physiologic concepts
   1. Intracranial pressure (ICP) is determined by the components within the cranial vault: brain tissue volume, cerebrospinal fluid (CSF), and blood volume
   2. ICP is dynamic
      a. It varies with arterial pulsations, respirations, and such activities as coughing and sneezing
      b. The Monro-Kellie hypothesis states that when the volume of one component increases, the total pressure will increase unless a reciprocal change occurs in another component
   3. Compensation for increased ICP occurs through various means
      a. Displacement of CSF (most compensation occurs this way)
      b. Reduction of cerebral blood volume
      c. Displacement of brain tissue (HERNIATION OF THE BRAIN)
   4. Systemic arterial pressure and ICP affect cerebral perfusion
      a. Cerebral perfusion pressure (CPP) provides an estimate of cerebral blood flow; it is the difference between cerebral arterial and venous pressure
      b. CPP can be affected by changes in mean arterial pressure (MAP) or ICP
      c. MAP is the average pressure during a complete cardiac cycle, the period from the beginning of ventricular systole to the end of ventricular diastole; it is calculated by the following formula:

$$\text{MAP} = \frac{(2 \times \text{diastolic}) + \text{systolic}}{3}$$

      d. CPP is calculated by the formula CPP = MAP − ICP
      e. A mechanism termed autoregulation allows consistent cerebral blood flow, provided MAP is between 60 and 130 mm Hg
   5. ICP monitoring requires insertion of a sensor or catheter into a specific cranial area
   6. The three most commonly monitored cranial areas are the lateral ventricle, the subarachnoid space, and the EPIDURAL SPACE; because its usefulness is limited, epidural monitoring is the method used least frequently by major trauma centers

B. ICP monitoring requirements
   1. Informed consent must be secured
   2. Aseptic technique is essential during the insertion and maintenance of the monitoring device

CLINICAL ALERT

3. The system must be free of air to reproduce intracranial waveforms accurately
4. A continuous-flush device is contraindicated because infusion of fluid into the brain will increase ICP
5. The transducer is leveled at the FORAMEN OF MONRO
6. The monitor must be balanced and calibrated routinely, according to institutional policy
7. Variations in values should be regarded as trends

C. Uses
1. Helps prevent or minimize neurologic damage in a patient with a neurologic problem, such as head trauma (especially closed head injuries), ruptured cerebral aneurysm, Reye's syndrome, known or suspected hydrocephalus, and brain tumor
2. Allows for observation of trends and changes in a patient's condition
3. Indicates a change in ICP before other signs are clinically present

D. Normal readings
1. ICP ranges from 0 to 10 mm Hg, with an upper limit of 15 mm Hg
2. CPP is 80 to 90 mm Hg
3. Waveform appearance depends on the measurement method and associated pathology and can be affected by arterial pulsation, cerebral vasodilation, and changes in venous outflow; waveforms may resemble arterial pressure or central venous pressure waveforms

E. Implications of abnormal readings
1. If MAP decreases or ICP increases, CPP decreases
2. If CPP falls below 60 mm Hg, ischemia occurs within the brain
3. If MAP equals ICP, blood flow ceases within the brain
4. Waveform variations, known as A, B, or C waves, may occur
   a. *A waves* (plateau waves) are rapid, spontaneous, sustained increases in pressure, usually from 50 to 100 mm Hg but sometimes approaching 200 mm Hg, that last for 5 to 20 minutes before falling spontaneously; they indicate intracranial decompensation and compression
   b. *B waves* are sharp, small waves with pressure up to 50 mm Hg; they correspond to changes in respiration and may be caused by variations in cerebral blood volume
   c. *C waves* are small, rhythmic waves with pressures up to 20 mm Hg that occur at a rate of up to 6 per minute; they are related to pressure and, like A waves, indicate intracranial compression

F. Patient care management varies with the monitoring method; for a patient with a ventricular catheter or subarachnoid screw, do the following
1. Analyze pressure data for trends, which are more significant than any specific reading

2. Monitor CPP by the formula CPP = MAP − ICP
3. Assess for abnormal waveforms: A (plateau), B, or C waves; report A waves to the doctor because they are clinically significant
4. Maintain the transducer at the foramen of Monro (the external landmark is the outer canthus of the eye or the top of the ear) to ensure accurate readings
5. Maintain a fluid-filled pressure system; do not connect the monitoring device to a pressure bag or a continuous-infusion system
6. If the waveforms are decreased or dampened, flush the system only if institutional policy allows (do not aspirate the system to attempt to remove the obstruction)
7. Zero and calibrate the transducer with changes in readings, according to institutional policy
8. Maintain aseptic technique during insertion and maintenance to minimize the risk of infection
9. Check the system for leaks; use Luer-Lok connectors when possible
10. Change the transducer, tubing, and dressing according to institutional policy
11. Perform patient teaching about ICP (see *Patient undergoing ICP monitoring,* page 74)

♦ II. Intraventricular ICP monitoring

A. General information
1. The ventricular catheter usually is inserted through a drill hole made in the dura and into the anterior horn of the lateral ventricle in the nondominant hemisphere
2. Sometimes the catheter is inserted into the posterior horn of the lateral ventricle in the nondominant hemisphere
3. The procedure is performed with the patient under local anesthesia
4. The catheter is connected to a pressure transducer by a stopcock or pressure tubing

B. Advantages
1. Measures CSF pressure directly (most accurate method)
2. Therapeutically drains excess CSF
3. Allows for recalibration of the transducer
4. Offers the ability to test intracranial VOLUME PRESSURE RESPONSES (a measure of intracranial elastance and compliance)
5. Allows instillation of contrast media for testing

C. Disadvantages
1. Requires puncturing of the brain, increasing the risk of brain tissue damage
2. Increases risk of intracranial infection
3. Makes insertion difficult if the ventricles are small or displaced

TEACHING TIPS

Patient undergoing ICP monitoring

Be sure to include both the patient and family members in your teaching. Acknowledge their fears and answer all questions. Your teaching should cover the following topics.

- Basic facts about ICP monitoring and the type of device used
- Rationale for ICP monitoring and associated nursing activities
- Alarms and what they mean
- Signs and symptoms to report to the nurse
- The need for frequent monitoring of the patient's status and the effects of therapy

4. May cause excess loss of CSF
5. May be blocked by blood clots

♦ III. Subarachnoid screw monitoring

A. General information
1. A hollow screw is inserted through a burr hole made in the skull and into the subarachnoid space
2. The procedure is performed with the patient under local anesthesia
3. The catheter is connected to a pressure transducer by a stopcock or pressure tubing

B. Advantages
1. Measures CSF pressure directly
2. Therapeutically drains CSF
3. Allows for recalibration of the transducer

C. Disadvantages
1. Increases risk of intracranial infection
2. May cause excess loss of CSF
3. Does not allow instillation of contrast media
4. May be blocked by swelling brain tissue

♦ IV. Epidural monitoring

A. General information
1. An intracranial transducer or balloon is inserted between the skull and dura
2. The transducer or balloon is connected to an external monitor

B. Advantages
1. Poses less danger of infection than other methods
2. Monitors ICP without opening dura

C. Disadvantages
   1. May not reflect ICP accurately because epidural pressure is higher than intraventricular pressure
   2. Does not allow for draining of CSF
   3. Increases the possibility of inaccurate readings because some systems cannot be recalibrated
   4. Does not allow for testing of volume pressure responses

POINTS TO REMEMBER

- ICP is dynamic and affected by most activities of daily living.
- Systemic arterial pressure and ICP affect cerebral perfusion.
- The trend in data is more significant than any one reading.
- The most accurate method of ICP monitoring is the intraventricular method.

STUDY QUESTIONS

To evaluate your understanding of this chapter, answer the following questions in the space provided; then compare your responses with the correct answers in Appendix B, page 281.

1. What determines ICP? ______________________________

____

____

2. Where must the nurse maintain the transducer to ensure accurate readings?

____

____

3. What do C waves indicate? ______________________________

____

____

4. What are the advantages of epidural monitoring? ______________

____

____

CRITICAL THINKING AND APPLICATION EXERCISES

1. Observe and document the effects of hyperventilation on ICP readings in a patient undergoing ICP monitoring.
2. List five nursing interventions that will reduce ICP.
3. Work with a fellow student to develop a chart describing the advantages and disadvantages for each method of ICP monitoring.
4. Calculate CPP in a patient with a blood pressure of 90/60 and an ICP of 20 mm Hg. Discuss the patient care management indications.

CHAPTER

10

Continuous Cardiac Monitoring

Learning objectives

After studying this chapter, you should be able to:

- Describe the general principles for the patient requiring continuous cardiac monitoring.
- Identify the common leads used for cardiac monitoring.
- Discuss care management for a patient undergoing cardiac monitoring.
- Explain the significance of the normal electrocardiographic (ECG) waveforms, segments, and intervals.
- Identify the ECG characteristics of normal sinus rhythm.

Chapter overview

A basic component of critical care and emergency nursing, continuous cardiac monitoring allows for ongoing observation of the heart's electrical activity. Essential skills for cardiac continuous monitoring include correct electrode placement based on the selected monitoring lead and the ability to recognize a normal sinus rhythm, the waveform characteristic of the normal cardiac cycle. Normal sinus rhythm provides the standard for identifying all other rhythms.

♦ I. Introduction

A. Physiologic concepts
  1. Cardiac monitoring measures the heart's electrical activity, displayed as waveforms, by the placement of electrodes on the chest
    a. Each waveform represents a particular event in the cardiac cycle
    b. Waveforms are identified by the letters P, Q, R, S, and T
  2. The patient may be monitored continuously while in bed (hard-wire monitoring) or while ambulatory (TELEMETRY)
    a. Electrodes are placed on the chest to allow for patient mobility; they are not placed on bony prominences

CLINICAL ALERT

    b. The conductant used on the electrodes must be moist
    c. The quality of the electrocardiogram (ECG) waveform is dependent on the electrode conductant and the electrode placement

B. Basic monitoring equipment components
  1. OSCILLOSCOPE
  2. Alarms: controls that let the user set limits for fast or slow heart rates
  3. Hard copy: printout of ECG tracing on standardized graph paper

C. Rate and rhythm determination
  1. Rate and rhythm are determined from the monitor or hard copy
  2. Time is measured along the horizontal axis on the hard copy; each small block represents 0.04 second, and each large block represents 0.20 second
  3. The hard copy is usually marked at 3- to 6-second intervals
  4. The recording speed on the monitor and hard copy should be set at 25 mm/second so that 300 large blocks pass through the recorder each minute
  5. The rate may be obtained from a digital readout display or calculated from the hard copy by determining the number of cardiac cycles in a 6-second interval and multiplying by 10
  6. The rhythm may be determined on the hard copy by measuring the length between the R-R intervals (determines ventricular rhythm) or P-P intervals (determines atrial rhythm) using CALIPERS

D. Continuous monitoring uses
  1. To monitor cardiac rhythm in critically ill patients
  2. To observe symptomatic arrhythmias or cardiac pathology
  3. To evaluate drug, fluid, or electrolyte therapy

E. Cardiac monitoring limitations

CLINICAL ALERT

  1. Measures only electrical activity
  2. Is not an indicator of cardiac mechanical function
  3. Requires evaluation of and correlation with the patient's clinical status before any intervention for a cardiac rhythm identified by continuous cardiac monitoring is performed

TEACHING TIPS

Patient receiving continuous cardiac monitoring

Be sure to include the following topics when preparing your teaching plan for the patient receiving continuous cardiac monitoring.

- Rationale for monitoring
- Information obtained from the monitor
- Alarms and controls
- Lead placement, including the need for leads to stay in place
- Activity restrictions, if necessary
- Signs and symptoms to report

4. Is not a substitute for a 12-lead diagnostic ECG

F. Patient care management
1. Explain the procedure to the patient
2. Prepare the skin for electrode placement by shaving, cleaning, and abrading to decrease skin resistance to the transmission of electrical signals from the heart
3. Place the electrodes in the correct locations based on lead selection
4. Prevent artifact or electrical shock by grounding the equipment
5. Set the high- and low-rate alarms
6. Observe the monitor for changes in rate, rhythm, or conduction; document and report significant changes to the doctor
7. Document and report chest pain and diaphoresis to the doctor, especially if they occur concurrently with monitor changes
8. Perform patient teaching (see *Patient receiving continuous cardiac monitoring*)

♦ II. Types of leads

A. General information
1. Two common types of monitoring leads are LEAD II and MCL_1
2. Waveform deflection is determined by the lead selection

B. Lead II
1. Lead II produces *upright* waveform deflections; P waves are seen clearly
2. The positive electrode is placed at the left midclavicular line, at or below the fifth intercostal space
3. The negative electrode is placed on the right shoulder, below the clavicle
4. The ground electrode stabilizes the electrical pattern and may be placed at any location on the body

C. MCL_1

1. MCL_1 produces *inverted* waveform deflections
   a. It simulates the precordial V_1 lead of a 12-lead ECG
   b. It offers more diagnostic advantages for identifying ectopy and blocks
2. The positive electrode is placed at the fourth intercostal space, on the right sternal border
3. The negative electrode is placed on the left shoulder, below the clavicle
4. The ground electrode stabilizes the electrical pattern and may be placed at any location on the body

♦ III. Characteristics of a normal cardiac cycle

A. General information

1. Polarization and repolarization are the electrical events in a cardiac cycle
2. Each electrical event is represented by a deflection of a waveform

B. P wave

1. The P wave represents atrial depolarization and indicates sinoatrial node function
2. Location: precedes the QRS complex
3. Duration: 0.06 to 0.11 second
4. Configuration: usually symmetrically rounded and upright in lead II; may be diphasic (positive and negative), flat, or inverted in MCL_1

C. QRS complex

1. The QRS complex represents ventricular depolarization
2. Location: follows the PR interval
3. Duration: less than 0.10 second
4. Configuration: different in each lead; the Q wave is the first negative deflection (may not always appear); the R wave is the first positive deflection; the S wave is the negative deflection after the R wave

D. T wave

1. The T wave represents ventricular repolarization
2. Location: follows the S wave and ST segment
3. Duration: not usually measured
4. Configuration: usually rounded, upright, smooth, and less than 5 mm in lead II; direction of deflection in MCL_1 is variable

E. PR interval

1. The PR interval represents the time it takes the impulse to reach the Purkinje fibers

Normal cardiac cycle

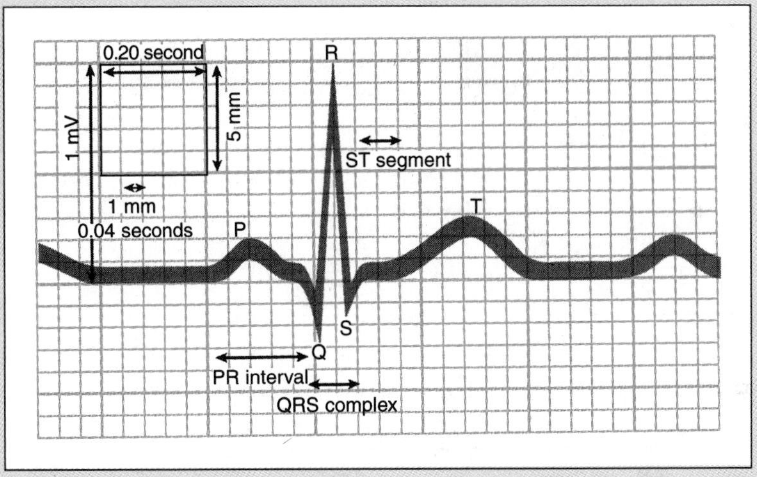

2. Location: extends from beginning of P wave to beginning of QRS complex
3. Duration: 0.12 to 0.20 second

F. ST segment
   1. The ST segment represents the end of ventricular depolarization and the beginning of repolarization
   2. Location: extends from end of S wave to beginning of T wave
   3. Duration: not usually measured
   4. Configuration: usually ISOELECTRIC, not varying more than 1 mm (one small vertical block)

G. Normal sinus rhythm
   1. Rhythm originating in the sinus node with all characteristics of a normal cardiac cycle (see *Normal cardiac cycle*)
   2. Rate ranges from 60 to 100 beats/minute

Points to remember

- Cardiac monitoring transforms the heart's electrical activity into a series of waveforms.
- Cardiac monitoring measures only cardiac electrical activity and is not an indicator of cardiac mechanical function.

- Each cardiac monitoring lead generates its own characteristic waveforms.
- The basic waveforms are the P wave, the QRS complex, and the T wave.

STUDY QUESTIONS

To evaluate your understanding of this chapter, answer the following questions in the space provided; then compare your responses with the correct answers in Appendix B, pages 281 and 282.

1. What are the major indications for cardiac monitoring? ______________

2. What are the major limitations to cardiac monitoring? ______________

3. Which monitoring lead produces upright waveforms and clear P waves?

4. Which monitoring lead produces inverted waveform deflections and is helpful in identifying ectopy and blocks? ______________

CRITICAL THINKING AND APPLICATION EXERCISES

1. Determine the standard monitoring leads used in the clinical setting.
2. Research your institution's procedure for continuous monitoring, including placement and changing of electrodes.
3. Obtain a rhythm strip from a patient on continuous cardiac monitoring, and identify each characteristic of the cardiac cycle.
4. Determine if your institution has telemetry monitoring, and describe how it differs from continuous cardiac monitoring.

CHAPTER

11

Cardiac Arrhythmias

Learning objectives

After studying this chapter, you should be able to:

- Discuss general principles of arrhythmia interpretation.
- Describe the electrocardiogram characteristics for each type of arrhythmia.
- Identify life-threatening arrhythmias.
- Describe care management for a patient with a life-threatening arrhythmia.

Chapter overview

All critical care and emergency nurses must learn to promptly and accurately identify cardiac arrhythmias. You can interpret any arrhythmia by using the five-step system described below. You will also find criteria for interpretation and therapeutic management for selected arrhythmias.

I. Introduction

A. Physiologic concepts
   1. ARRHYTHMIA is any disturbance in the normal rhythm of the heartbeat
   2. Disturbances or irregularities in rhythm occur because of alteration in automaticity, conductivity, or both

B. Interpretation
   1. Five steps are used to interpret arrhythmias
      a. Determine the rate (both atrial and ventricular)
      b. Determine the rhythm (regular or irregular)
      c. Analyze the P waves (normal, with one for each QRS complex)
      d. Measure the P-R interval (intervals outside the normal range indicate a conduction disturbance)
      e. Measure the duration of the QRS complex (a duration longer than normal indicates a ventricular conduction disturbance)
   2. Arrhythmia interpretation may require analysis of the rhythm in more than one lead (for examples of selected arrhythmias, see the appendix Identifying and Treating Arrhythmias)

C. Classification of arrhythmias
   1. Arrhythmias are classified according to site
      a. Sinus
      b. Atrial
      c. Junctional
      d. Ventricular
      e. Atrioventricular (AV)
   2. Rhythms of undetermined origin (initiated at a site above the ventricles) are called supraventricular

II. Sinus bradycardia

A. Definition: arrhythmia in which all impulses originate in the sinus node, but the rate is less than 60 beats/minute

B. Electrocardiogram (ECG) characteristics
   1. Rate: less than 60 beats/minute for atrial and ventricular rates
   2. Rhythm: regular; atrial and ventricular are the same
   3. P wave: normal
   4. PR interval: within normal limits
   5. QRS complex: within normal limits
   6. ST segment: normal
   7. T wave: normal

C. Possible causes: exercise or sleep (may be normal), sedation, increased intracranial pressure, increased vagal tone from straining or vomiting,

TEACHING TIPS

Patient with an arrhythmia

Be sure to include the following topics when preparing your teaching plan for the patient with an arrhythmia.

- Type of arrhythmia and its underlying cause
- Signs and symptoms and associated complications
- Treatment
- Medication therapy, if ordered
- Basic cardiac life support measures
- Medical follow-up

mechanical ventilation, sick sinus syndrome, hypothyroidism, hyperkalemia, and drug therapy with beta blockers or sympatholytics

D. Clinical significance depends on the cause and symptoms

E. Patient care management
1. Do not intervene if the patient is asymptomatic
2. Treat the underlying cause (see *Patient with an arrhythmia*)

♦ III. Sinus tachycardia

A. Definition: arrhythmia in which all impulses originate in the sinus node, but the rate is accelerated

B. ECG characteristics
1. Rate: atrial and ventricular rates are 100 to 160 beats/minute
2. Rhythm: regular; atrial and ventricular are the same
3. P wave: normal but may not be visible if the rate exceeds 140 beats/minute
4. PR interval: within normal limits
5. QRS complex: within normal limits
6. ST segment: normal
7. T wave: normal

C. Possible causes: normal physiologic response to the demand for increased oxygen during stress or activity; caffeine, nicotine, or alcohol; pain; such drugs as adrenergics, anticholinergics, and some antiarrhythmics; digitalis toxicity; decrease in vagal tone and increase in sympathetic tone; hyperthyroidism; and anemia, hypovolemia, or hypotension

D. Clinical significance
1. None if it is a normal response
2. Increased rate increases myocardial oxygen demand and can lead to ischemia and myocardial damage

E. Patient care management
   1. Treat the underlying cause
   2. Observe the patient for signs and symptoms of hypoxia and congestive heart failure (CHF)
   3. Have patient perform Valsalva's maneuver or cough for vagal nerve stimulation. Doctor may do carotid sinus massage

CLINICAL ALERT

   4. Be aware that carotid massage is done only by a doctor after determining that the patient does not have a carotid bruit because massage could result in embolization of a stenotic plaque in the carotid artery, causing a stroke

♦ IV. Atrial fibrillation

A. Definition: 400 to 500 unorganized ectopic impulses per minute in the atria, producing atrial quiver instead of contraction

B. ECG characteristics
   1. Rate: atrial rate is indiscernible; ventricular rate is usually 100 to 150 beats/minute
   2. Rhythm: atrial and ventricular grossly irregular
   3. P wave: none
   4. PR interval: indiscernible
   5. QRS complex: within normal limits
   6. ST segment: unidentifiable
   7. T wave: unidentifiable

C. Possible causes: valvular disease, coronary artery disease (CAD), cardiomyopathy, myocardial infarction (MI), constrictive pericarditis, CHF, chronic obstructive pulmonary disease (COPD), thyrotoxicosis, and increased sympathetic activity

D. Clinical significance
   1. Cardiac output may be decreased by as much as 30%
   2. Mural thrombi may develop in the atria and migrate to the pulmonary or systemic circulation, causing a pulmonary or peripheral embolus

E. Patient care management
   1. Administer digitalis, verapamil, or beta blockers to increase AV node refractoriness or quinidine or procainamide to prolong atrial refractoriness
   2. Have patient perform Valsalva's maneuver or cough, which may reduce the rapid ventricular rate (if atrial fibrillation is not chronic)
   3. Administer anticoagulants to decrease clot formation

4. Deliver synchronized CARDIOVERSION according to advanced cardiac life support (ACLS) protocols if the patient is hemodynamically unstable
5. Treat the underlying cause to prevent recurrence

♦ V. Atrial flutter

A. Definition: arrhythmia characterized by a rapid atrial rate of 250 to 350 beats/minute

B. ECG characteristics
1. Rate: atrial rate may be 250 to 350 beats/minute; ventricular rate depends on degree of AV block, usually 60 to 100 beats/minute; the ratio of atrial to ventricular conduction may be 1:2, 1:3, or 1:4
2. Rhythm: atrial and ventricular are usually regular
3. P wave: saw-toothed flutter waves; two, three, or four for each QRS complex
4. PR interval: usually not measurable
5. QRS complex: usually within normal limits
6. ST segment: unidentifiable
7. T wave: unidentifiable

C. Possible causes: MI, valvular disease, cor pulmonale, pericarditis, digitalis toxicity, hyperthyroidism, pulmonary embolism, and postoperative revascularization

D. Clinical significance
1. Depends on the ventricular rate
2. More difficult to convert than atrial fibrillation

E. Patient care management
1. Administer verapamil, digitalis (unless the condition is caused by digitalis toxicity), or propranolol
2. Administer quinidine, which may convert flutter to fibrillation
3. Deliver synchronized cardioversion according to ACLS protocols if the ventricular rate is rapid and patient is hemodynamically unstable

♦ VI. Supraventricular tachycardia

A. Definition: arrhythmia with rate greater than 100 beats/minute originating above the ventricle but not in the sinoatrial (SA) node
1. Atrial tachycardia: impulses originate in the atria at rates of 150 to 250 beats/minute
2. Reentry pathway: impulses originate at the AV node often after a premature beat

3. Paroxysmal: starting and stopping abruptly
   a. Paroxysmal supraventricular tachycardia
   b. Paroxysmal atrial tachycardia

B. ECG characteristics
1. Rate: atrial rate greater than 140 beats/minute; ventricular rate depends on degree of block
2. Rhythm: atrial and ventricular usually regular, starting and stopping abruptly; may be irregular if impulses originate from multifocal areas
3. P wave: upright, regular, but aberrant; may not be visible or may be difficult to distinguish from preceding T wave
4. PR interval: usually not measurable
5. QRS complex: usually within normal limits
6. ST segment: unidentifiable
7. T wave: unidentifiable

C. Possible causes: physical or psychological stress; hypoxia; hypokalemia; caffeine, other stimulants, or marijuana; MI; chronic lung disease; congenital heart disease; and hyperthyroidism

D. Clinical significance
1. Benign in healthy people
2. May precede more serious ventricular arrhythmias when it occurs with cardiac or pulmonary disease

E. Patient care management
1. Have patient perform Valsalva's maneuver or cough for vagal nerve stimulation to slow AV node conduction
2. Administer drug therapy, which may include adenosine, digitalis, propranolol, or verapamil
3. Deliver synchronized cardioversion according to ACLS protocols if the patient is hemodynamically unstable
4. Consider atrial overdrive pacing
5. Treat the underlying cause

♦ VII. First-degree AV block

A. Definition: conduction disturbance in which the electrical impulses are delayed at the AV node

B. ECG characteristics
1. Rate: atrial and ventricular rates are equal at 60 to 100 beats/minute
2. Rhythm: atrial and ventricular regular
3. P wave: normal
4. PR interval: prolonged more than 0.20 second but constant
5. QRS complex: usually within normal limits

6. ST segment: normal
7. T wave: normal

C. Possible causes: such drugs as quinidine, procainamide, digitalis, and propranolol; rheumatic fever; chronic degeneration of the conduction system; potassium imbalance; myocardial ischemia; MI; and hypothyroidism

D. Clinical significance: none

E. Patient care management
1. Monitor carefully for AV block progressing to higher degree
2. Withhold any drug that may be the cause
3. Do not intervene if the patient is asymptomatic

♦ VIII. Second-degree AV block, Mobitz type I

A. Definition: conduction disturbance in which the AV node conducts each successive impulse earlier and earlier until an impulse arrives during the absolute refractory period and cannot be conducted

B. ECG characteristics
1. Rate: atrial rate is greater than ventricular but both are usually within normal limits
2. Rhythm: atrial is regular; ventricular is irregular because of progressive shortening of the R-R interval
3. P wave: normal
4. PR interval: lengthens progressively with each cycle until a P wave appears without a QRS complex
5. QRS complex: normal but is dropped periodically
6. ST segment: within normal limits
7. T wave: normal

C. Possible causes: inferior wall MI, digitalis toxicity, acute rheumatic fever, electrolyte imbalance, and drug therapy with quinidine or procainamide

D. Clinical significance
1. Prognosis is good if the patient is asymptomatic
2. Second-degree AV block may progress to a more serious block
3. Second-degree, type I AV block is also referred to as Wenkebach block

E. Patient care management
1. Treat the underlying cause
2. Use atropine or prepare the symptomatic patient for insertion of a temporary pacemaker

♦ IX. Second-degree AV block, Mobitz type II

A. Definition: conduction disturbance in which dropped beats occur without warning; the abnormality is in the bundle of His or the bundle branches

B. ECG characteristics
1. Rate: atrial is usually within normal limits; ventricular is slower
2. Rhythm: atrial is regular; ventricular may be irregular
3. P wave: normal
4. PR interval: within normal limits or prolonged but always constant
5. QRS complex: normal but periodically absent
6. ST segment: normal unless myocardial ischemia or damage is present
7. T wave: normal

C. Possible causes: anterior wall MI, severe CAD, and other organic heart disease

D. Clinical significance
1. More serious than Mobitz type I because it is unpredictable
2. May progress to third-degree (complete) heart block

E. Patient care management
1. Administer vasoactive drugs to maintain blood pressure and cardiac output
2. Prepare the patient for insertion of a temporary pacemaker to stabilize hemodynamic status
3. Prepare the patient for insertion of a permanent pacemaker to prevent ventricular standstill

CLINICAL ALERT

4. Carefully monitor patients with diagnosed AV conduction defects (blocks of any degree) for progression to a higher degree of block, as indicated by change in heart rate, rhythm, or length of PR interval or QRS duration or configuration

♦ X. Third-degree AV block (complete heart block)

A. Definition: condition in which all atrial impulses are blocked at the AV junction and a secondary pacemaker (in the junction or ventricle) stimulates the ventricles; the atria and ventricles beat independently

B. ECG characteristics
1. Rate: atrial is faster than ventricular, which is usually less than 45 beats/minute
2. Rhythm: atrial has regular P-P intervals and ventricular has regular R-R intervals, but no relation exists between atrial and ventricular rhythms
3. P wave: normal

4. PR interval: inapplicable because the atria and ventricles beat independently of each other; may appear to vary
5. QRS complex: configuration depends on origin of ventricular stimulus; may be narrow, wide, or bizarre
6. ST segment: normal
7. T wave: normal

C. Possible causes: anterior wall MI, acute digitalis toxicity, postoperative complication of mitral or aortic valve replacement, rheumatic fever, and congenital abnormalities

D. Clinical significance
1. Slow ventricular rates decrease cardiac output
2. Ventricular arrhythmias may develop if a secondary pacemaker in the ventricle becomes irritable
3. Failure of a ventricular pacemaker results in cardiac arrest

E. Patient care management: see "Patient care management," page 90

♦ XI. Left bundle-branch block (LBBB)

A. Definition: conduction delay in the left posterior and anterior branches of the left bundle that disrupts normal left-to-right ventricular activation; an incomplete LBBB represents an altered conduction in either the posterior or the anterior branch

B. ECG characteristics
1. Rate: atrial and ventricular within normal limits
2. Rhythm: atrial and ventricular regular
3. P wave: normal
4. PR interval: within normal limits
5. QRS complex: complete LBBB shows duration of 0.12 second or greater; incomplete LBBB shows duration between 0.10 and 0.12 second (deflection of the QRS complex varies with lead selection)
6. ST segment: usually abnormal in size and configuration and occurs in opposite direction of QRS complex
7. T wave: deflection is in opposite direction of QRS complex in most leads

C. Possible causes: MI, hypertension, CAD, myocarditis, valvular disease, congenital abnormalities, ventricular hypertrophy, and degenerative diseases of the cardiac conduction system

D. Clinical significance
1. Usually does not occur in healthy people
2. Indicates underlying heart disease
3. LBBB with left axis deviation associated with higher morbidity and mortality

E. Patient care management
   1. Usually none is required for the block itself
   2. Prepare the patient for insertion of a pacemaker (if it is required to treat LBBB with acute anteroseptal MI)
   3. Treat the underlying cause

♦ XII. Right bundle-branch block (RBBB)

A. Definition: conduction delay in the right bundle branch
   1. It causes the right ventricle to be activated late
   2. Depolarizing forces spread through the system from the left ventricle instead of almost simultaneously with the left ventricle

B. ECG characteristics
   1. Rate: atrial and ventricular within normal limits
   2. Rhythm: atrial and ventricular regular
   3. P wave: normal
   4. PR interval: within normal limits
   5. QRS complex: complete RBBB shows duration of 0.12 second or greater; incomplete RBBB shows duration between 0.10 and 0.12 second (deflection of the QRS complex varies with lead selection)
   6. ST segment: usually abnormal and occurs in opposite direction of QRS complex
   7. T wave: deflection is in opposite direction of QRS complex

C. Possible causes: acute heart failure, CAD, MI, hypokalemia, digitalis toxicity, valvular or congenital anomalies, right ventricular hypertrophy, acute pulmonary embolism, atherosclerosis of the conduction system, and right-sided cardiac catheterization

D. Clinical significance: aids in diagnosis of other conditions

E. Patient care management
   1. Usually none is required for the block itself
   2. Prepare the patient for insertion of a pacemaker (if it is required to treat RBBB with acute anteroseptal MI)
   3. Treat the underlying cause

♦ XIII. Premature atrial contraction

A. Definition: beat that originates outside the SA node, usually because of an irritable focus in the atria

B. ECG characteristics
   1. Rate: atrial and ventricular usually within normal limits
   2. Rhythm: atrial and ventricular irregular because of the premature beat; underlying rhythm may be regular
   3. P wave: premature and abnormal in the premature beat
   4. PR interval: longer or shorter than normal in the premature beat

5. QRS complex: usually within normal limits in the premature beat
6. ST segment: normal
7. T wave: normal or may be distorted if the P wave is early

C. Possible causes: CHF, CAD, valvular heart disease, COPD, hypoxia, stress, fatigue, and caffeine, tobacco, or alcohol

D. Clinical significance
1. Rarely dangerous in the patient without heart disease
2. May precipitate more serious arrhythmia, such as atrial fibrillation or flutter
3. May indicate CHF or electrolyte imbalance

E. Patient care management
1. Monitor for signs and symptoms of heart failure
2. Administer drug therapy, which may include digitalis, verapamil, or quinidine
3. Eliminate caffeine, tobacco, and alcohol

♦ XIV. Premature ventricular contraction (PVC)

A. Definition: ectopic beat originating from a stimulus in the ventricles that occurs earlier than the normally expected beat and that is usually followed by a compensatory pause

B. ECG characteristics
1. Rate: atrial and ventricular usually within normal limits but may be slow if many PVCs are present
2. Rhythm: atrial and ventricular irregular because of the PVCs, but the underlying rhythm may be regular
3. P wave: absent in the premature beat unless retrograde conduction is present; then the P wave may follow the QRS complex
4. PR interval: absent in the premature beat
5. QRS complex: wider than 0.12 second and bizarre because the impulse arises from the ventricle in the premature beat
6. ST segment: not considered because of abnormal depolarization of ventricles
7. T wave: deflection is in the opposite direction of the widened QRS complex and is followed by a long compensatory pause in the premature beat

C. Possible causes: digitalis toxicity; hypokalemia; hypocalcemia; hypoxia; caffeine, tobacco, or alcohol ingestion; sympathomimetic drugs, such as epinephrine and isoproterenol; irritation of the myocardium by pacemaker electrodes; and exercise above normal tolerance levels

D. Clinical significance
  1. Decreased cardiac output because of a PVC
  2. In ischemic heart disease, PVCs are more likely to stimulate ventricular tachycardia, flutter, or fibrillation

CLINICAL ALERT

  3. Dangerous forms include two or more in a row, BIGEMINY (every other beat is a PVC), multifocal (more than one irritable foci), more than six occurring in 1 minute, and R-ON-T PHENOMENON

E. Patient care management
  1. Do not treat if PVCs are rare and patient is otherwise healthy
  2. Administer oxygen if hypoxia is the cause
  3. Administer electrolyte replacement if imbalance is the cause
  4. Administer atropine if rhythm is bradycardic
  5. Administer antiarrhythmics, such as lidocaine, to decrease irritability

CLINICAL ALERT

  6. Be aware that potassium levels within the range of 3.5 to 5.5 must be maintained to decrease the cardiac irritability and PVCs; hypokalemia and digoxin administration can result in increased arrhythmias

♦ XV. Ventricular tachycardia

A. Definition: more than three PVCs occurring in succession at a rate of more than 100 beats/minute

B. ECG characteristics
  1. Rate: atrial cannot be determined; ventricular is usually more rapid (100 to 250 beats/minute)
  2. Rhythm: atrial cannot be determined; ventricular is usually regular or slightly irregular
  3. P wave: usually not visible but may be retrograde
  4. PR interval: cannot be identified
  5. QRS complex: wide and bizarre; may resemble PVCs recorded before tachycardia began
  6. ST segment: difficult or impossible to determine
  7. T wave: deflection in the opposite direction of QRS complex

C. Possible causes: myocardial ischemia, MI, rheumatic heart disease, mitral valve prolapse, CHF, cardiomyopathy, pulmonary embolism, electrolyte imbalance, and drug toxicity from digitalis, procainamide, quinidine, or epinephrine

D. Clinical significance
  1. Life-threatening
  2. May deteriorate to ventricular fibrillation

E. Patient care management
  1. Do not plan to treat asymptomatic bursts of ventricular tachycardia that spontaneously convert

2. Administer antiarrhythmics to decrease ventricular irritability
3. If the patient is hemodynamically unstable, defibrillate immediately with 200 joules followed by a second DEFIBRILLATION of 200 to 300 joules and a third defibrillation of 360 joules, if necessary
4. Initiate basic cardiac life support (BCLS) and ACLS protocols according to institutional policy
5. Prepare the patient for overdrive pacing, which may be considered if bradycardia is a causative factor
6. Prepare the patient for implantation of an automatic defibrillator, which may be considered if the patient does not respond to drug therapy

♦ XVI. Ventricular fibrillation

A. Definition: rapid, disorganized depolarization of the ventricles, characterized by a lack of specific electrical impulse, conduction, and contraction

B. ECG characteristics
1. Rate: cannot be determined
2. Rhythm: rapid and chaotic with no pattern or regularity
3. P wave: not identifiable
4. PR interval: not identifiable
5. QRS complex: not identifiable
6. ST segment: not identifiable
7. T wave: not identifiable

C. Possible causes: MI, untreated ventricular tachycardia, electrolyte imbalance, electric shock, hypothermia, and R-on-T phenomenon

D. Clinical significance: cardiac output stops and death follows quickly

E. Patient care management
1. Defibrillate immediately with 200 joules followed by a second defibrillation of 200 to 300 joules and a third defibrillation of 360 joules, if necessary
2. Initiate BCLS and ACLS protocols according to institutional policy

♦ XVII. Asystole (ventricular standstill)

A. Definition: total absence of ventricular electrical activity

B. ECG characteristics
1. Rate: atrial usually indiscernible but could be present within normal limits; ventricular indiscernible
2. Rhythm: atrial and ventricular usually indiscernible
3. P wave: may be present
4. PR interval: not measurable
5. QRS complex: absent

6. ST segment: absent
7. T wave: absent

C. Possible causes: acute respiratory failure, severe metabolic deficit, and extensive myocardial damage from ischemia, infarction, rupture, or aneurysm

D. Clinical significance
1. Life-threatening
2. Least responsive of lethal arrhythmias

E. Patient care management
1. Initiate BCLS and ACLS protocols according to institutional policy
2. Defibrillate if unable to distinguish asystole from fine ventricular fibrillation

CLINICAL ALERT

3. Fine ventricular fibrillation is more responsive to treatment than asystole; treat aggressively until the rhythm is identified as asystole or the patient does not respond to defibrillation
4. Prepare the patient for insertion of a temporary pacemaker

Points to remember

- Digitalis toxicity should be considered as a possible cause for arrhythmia in any patient taking the drug.
- Dangerous forms of PVCs include two or more in a row, bigeminy, multifocal, more than six in 1 minute, and R-on-T phenomenon.
- Immediate defibrillation is indicated for unstable ventricular tachycardia or ventricular fibrillation.
- BCLS and ACLS protocols should be implemented according to institutional policy for all life-threatening arrhythmias.

Study questions

To evaluate your understanding of this chapter, answer the following questions in the space provided; then compare your responses with the correct answers in Appendix B, page 282.

1. What three mechanisms cause arrhythmias? ______________________________

____

____

2. What are the five steps used to interpret arrhythmias? ____________

3. How are arrhythmias classified? ____________

4. What are common causes of bradycardia? ____________

5. What are common causes of tachycardia? ____________

6. Which AV blocks require insertion of a permanent pacemaker? ____________

7. What are the ECG waveform characteristics of a PVC? ____________

8. Which arrhythmias are considered to be life-threatening? ____________

CRITICAL THINKING AND APPLICATION EXERCISES

1. Ask an experienced nurse to assist you in using calipers to measure the PR interval and the QRS complex on an ECG.
2. Collect ECG rhythm strips of at least 10 of the rhythms described in this chapter, and evaluate the characteristics of each.
3. Explain the significance of R-on-T phenomenon to another nurse or classmate.
4. Determine which types of temporary pacemakers are available in the clinical setting and their indications for use.

CHAPTER

12

Alternative Management Therapies

Learning objectives

After studying this chapter, you should be able to:

- ♦ List the commonly used alternative management therapies in cardiac care.
- ♦ Discuss the uses for each therapy.
- ♦ Identify the complications associated with each type of therapy.
- ♦ Describe the patient care management for each type of therapy.

Chapter overview

Commonly used alternative management therapies in cardiac care improve the quality of life for patients with electrical or mechanical cardiac dysfunction. These therapies include pacemakers, implantable cardiac defibrillators, intra-aortic balloon pumps, and ventricular-assist devices. Each type of therapy has specific uses and complications associated with it. Critical care and emergency nurses usually are responsible for assessing the function of these devices, detecting associated complications, and helping the patient and family adjust to the changes resulting from alternative therapy.

♦ I. Introduction

A. Technological advances
   1. Technological advances in cardiac care have enhanced the ability to help patients with electrical or mechanical cardiac dysfunction and to improve their quality of life
   2. Alternative management therapies may be temporary or permanent
   3. Complications may result from immobility and restricted physical activity during therapy
   4. Commonly used alternative therapies include pacemakers, automatic implantable cardiac defibrillators, intra-aortic balloon pumps, and ventricular-assist devices
   5. Critical care and emergency nurses usually are responsible for assessing the function of these devices, detecting associated complications, and helping the patient and family adjust to the changes resulting from alternative therapy

B. Potential nursing diagnoses for a patient requiring the use of alternative management therapies
   1. Risk for injury
   2. Risk for infection
   3. Decreased cardiac output
   4. Sensory or perceptual alterations (auditory and visual)
   5. Impaired physical mobility
   6. Ineffective individual coping
   7. Ineffective family coping

♦ II. Cardiac pacing

A. General information
   1. Cardiac pacing provides an extrinsic electrical impulse to initiate depolarization of the myocardium
   2. A pacemaker can be used to regulate blood flow in the atrium, ventricle, or both (atrioventricular [AV] sequential)
   3. Cardiac pacing can be temporary or permanent

B. Equipment
   1. The pulse generator (pacemaker) is the power source run by batteries
   2. Lead wires are attached to a pulse generator and have one (unipolar) or two (bipolar) electrodes at the other end that are in contact with the endocardium
   3. A pacing artifact spike appears on the electrocardiogram (ECG) before the depolarization waveform

C. Types
  1. Temporary pacemakers are inserted by one of three routes
     a. *Transvenous:* placed in contact with the endocardium through a major vein by way of a percutaneous stick or cutdown
     b. EPICARDIAL: attached to the epicardium during cardiac surgery with the wires brought out through the skin in the mediastinal area
     c. *External:* anterior and posterior conducting pads are placed on the skin
  2. Permanent pacemakers are attached to the endocardium under fluoroscopy through the transvenous approach; the generator is implanted under the patient's skin
  3. Often programmable, permanent pacemaker settings can be readjusted noninvasively

D. Modes of pacing
  1. Modes of pacing determine how sensitive the pacemaker is to the patient's heartbeat; synchronous pacing is the most common mode
     a. Synchronous mode pacing (DEMAND MODE PACING) senses the patient's heart rate and emits an electrical impulse only if the patient's rate falls below a preset rate
     b. Asynchronous (fixed rate) mode pacing discharges an impulse at a preset rate, regardless of the patient's heart rate
  2. Pacemaker settings include rate, energy output, stimulation threshold, and sensitivity control

E. Coding system
  1. A coding system of pacemaker functioning has been developed by the Inter-Society Commission on Heart Disease Resources (see *Understanding pacemaker codes*)
  2. The first three letters of the code describe the basic pacemaker function
     a. The first letter refers to the chamber of the heart that is paced
     b. The second letter refers to the chamber that is sensed
     c. The third letter indicates the response to the sensed event

F. Uses
  1. Cardiac pacing is used to regulate the heart rate in patients with one of several cardiac problems
     a. SICK SINUS SYNDROME
     b. Symptomatic bradyarrhythmias
     c. AV block
     d. Second-degree AV block, types I and II
     e. Third-degree AV block
     f. Postcardiac surgery
     g. Ventricular overdrive pacing

Understanding pacemaker codes

The chart below identifies the Inter-Society Commission on Heart Disease Resources system of coding for pacemakers. This coding system explains the functioning of the pacemaker.

FUNCTION	CODE
Chamber paced	V = ventricle A = atrium D = dual 0 = none
Chamber sensed	V = ventricle A = atrium D = dual 0 = none
Response to sensing	T = triggers pacing I = inhibits pacing D = dual (triggers and inhibits pacing) 0 = none
Programmable functions	P = programmable rate or output M = multiprogrammability of rate, output, sensitivity, and so forth C = communicating functions (telemetry) R = rate modulation 0 = none
Antitachyarrhythmia functions	P = pacing (antitachyarrhythmia) S = shock D = dual (P and S) 0 = none

Adapted with permission from Bernstein, A.D., et al. "The generic pacemaker code for antibradyarrhythmia and adoptive-rate pacing and antitachyarrhythmia devices," *PACE* 10:795, 1987.

2. The goal is to maintain a safe cardiac rate that can sustain an adequate cardiac output (CO)

G. Complications
   1. Complications resulting from pacemaker insertion
      a. Local or systemic infection
      b. Pneumothorax (particularly with subclavical insertion)
      c. Perforation of the myocardium
      d. Arrhythmias
   2. Complications associated with the pacemaker system
      a. Failure to pace, as indicated by absence of pacemaker spike on ECG at anticipated time

b. Failure to sense, as indicated by inability to recognize patient's beats in the synchronous mode
c. Failure to capture, as indicated by absence of myocardial contraction after pacing spike

CLINICAL ALERT

d. Environmental interference, which may disrupt pacemaker function

H. Patient care management (temporary pacing)
1. Monitor ECG to document functioning of the pacemaker
2. Assess and document vital signs, level of consciousness, heart and lung sounds, urine output, and any signs or symptoms indicating changes in these parameters
3. Compare the rate, energy output, and sensitivity controls with those ordered by the doctor; settings should be included in the patient's plan of care
4. Keep plastic cover on setting dials to prevent accidental changes in settings
5. Make sure all equipment around patient is grounded
6. Wear rubber gloves when adjusting electrodes
7. Observe for signs of rhythmic hiccuping or diaphragmatic twitching, which may indicate perforation of the right ventricle by the electrode
8. If a pacing problem occurs, ensure that the pacemaker is on, the batteries are working, the dials are properly set, the connectors are secure, and the catheter has not been inadvertently pulled out; placing the patient in the left lateral position may be helpful in reestablishing contact of the lead wire with the endocardium if capturing is a problem
9. If the patient experiences cardiac arrest, make sure pacemaker is on, turn up rate to at least 60 beats/minute, and adjust stimulation threshold high enough to capture
10. If the patient needs to be defibrillated, refer to the manufacturer's recommendations on whether the pacemaker should be disconnected or turned off

I. Patient care management (permanent pacing)
1. Monitor ECG to document functioning of the pacemaker
2. Assess and document vital signs, level of consciousness, heart and lung sounds, urine output, and any signs or symptoms indicating changes in these parameters
3. Teach the patient to recognize signs and symptoms that necessitate medical attention (dizziness, fainting, prolonged fatigue, peripheral swelling, palpitations, shortness of breath, signs of infection at surgical site)

4. Teach the patient and family to check pulse daily for 1 minute; if the rate slows more than 5 beats/minute, the patient should recheck his pulse
5. Instruct the patient and family to notify the doctor if the slow rate continues

CLINICAL ALERT

6. Encourage the patient to carry medical identification that includes his name, the type of pacemaker, and the name and telephone number of his doctor

♦ III. Implantable cardiac defibrillator (ICD)

A. General information
1. In most patients with sudden cardiac death, the primary mechanism is presumed to be ventricular fibrillation (see Chapter 11)
2. The ICD, composed of a pulse generator and a lead system, is used to correct lethal ventricular arrhythmias
3. The ICD continuously analyzes a patient's cardiac rhythm and intervenes when ventricular fibrillation or tachycardia occurs in an attempt to terminate the arrhythmia; the device will not discharge if the arrhythmia terminates spontaneously
4. New tiered-therapy generators incorporate antitachycardia pacing (used as the first-line treatment for ventricular tachycardia before low-energy cardioversion), low-energy cardioversion (for ventricular tachycardia not responding to antitachycardia pacing), high-energy defibrillation (if rhythm deteriorates to ventricular fibrillation), and bradycardia backup pacing (if rhythm deteriorates to asystole or a slow idioventricular rhythm)
5. The ICD is surgically inserted through a medial sternotomy, lateral thoracotomy, or transvenous approach
   a. With the medial sternotomy or lateral thoracotomy approach, epicardial patch leads (the defibrillating electrodes) are sutured to the ventricular wall, two UNIPOLAR LEADS are attached to the epicardium as rate-sensing leads, and the pulse generator is placed in a pocket under the patient's skin
   b. With a transvenous approach, electrodes are placed in contact with the endocardium; with some models, an additional subcutaneous patch may be used to enhance defibrillation
6. The ICD will discharge up to five shocks when the programmed rate cutoff limit is reached
7. The ICD also stores and retrieves shock information
8. The ICD generator will last about 3 to 5 years before replacement is required

TEACHING TIPS
Patient with an ICD

Be sure to include the following topics in your teaching plan for the patient with an ICD.
- Rationale for the device
- What to expect if arrhythmias recur
- Transport by ambulance to the hospital if ICD fires
- Report of number of ICD discharges
- Environmental factors that may interfere with ICD function
- Activity limitations
- Need for a home defibrillator in case the ICD fails to convert the arrhythmia at home
- Family training by the manufacturer's representative before the patient goes home
- Signs and symptoms of complications, such as infection

9. In an emergency, defibrillation or cardioversion can be performed without damage to the ICD

B. Uses
1. The ICD is recommended for use in patients who have had one of the following cardiac problems
    a. An episode of cardiac arrest presumed to be caused by hemodynamically unstable tachyarrhythmias not associated with acute myocardial infarction
    b. Sustained ventricular tachycardia of unknown cause that has not responded to electrophysiologic testing
    c. Sustained ventricular tachycardia that has not responded to antiarrhythmic medications
2. The goal is to terminate lethal ventricular arrhythmias to prevent sudden cardiac death

C. Complications
1. Infection
2. Cardiac tamponade
3. Thromboembolism

D. Patient care management
1. Assess and document continuous ECG rhythm, vital signs, mental status, heart and lung sounds, urine output, and any signs or symptoms indicating changes in these parameters
2. If arrhythmias occur during hospitalization, document the ICD response

CLINICAL ALERT

3. Keep in mind that advanced cardiac life support should be instituted if the ICD does not successfully convert the arrhythmia (see Chapter 6)
4. Remember that most patients with an ICD continue to take antiarrhythmic medication, but the dosage may be decreased
5. Refer family to appropriate sources for cardiopulmonary resuscitation (CPR) training; family should initiate CPR if the patient experiences cardiac arrest and should not wait for the ICD to fire (for specific teaching tips, see *Patient with an ICD*)
6. Ensure that family can activate the emergency medical system if problems should occur at home

♦ IV. Intra-aortic balloon pump (IABP)

A. General information

1. The IABP is a counterpulsation device that assists the failing heart by decreasing oxygen demand through decreasing myocardial workload, increasing coronary artery perfusion, and reducing afterload
2. The IABP is a temporary measure that augments CO by up to 15%
3. The size of the balloon used varies according to the size of the patient; the average balloon in adults holds 30 to 40 cc of air
4. The balloon is commonly inserted through the femoral artery and is placed in the descending thoracic aorta distal to the subclavian artery
5. Using the QRS complex of the ECG as its trigger, the balloon inflates during diastole and deflates just before systole
6. Timing of the balloon pump is performed using the arterial waveform or ECG at the IABP console
7. Inflation of the balloon displaces blood in the aorta up into the coronary arteries and the major vessels of the head and downward to the renal arteries, enhancing arterial perfusion (diastolic augmentation)
8. Deflation of the balloon immediately before systole reduces the amount of pressure that must be overcome to eject blood from the ventricle, thereby decreasing myocardial oxygen consumption (afterload reduction)
9. As heart rate or rhythm changes, the nurse may need to adjust the timing of the balloon
10. The goal is to provide sufficient CO that supports adequate tissue perfusion while allowing the heart to rest and recover from the insult

B. Uses

1. Cardiogenic shock or heart failure
2. Failure to wean from cardiopulmonary bypass during coronary artery bypass graft surgery
3. Elective preoperative placement in high-risk patients
4. Unstable angina that does not respond to conventional therapy
5. Refractory ventricular arrhythmias
6. Support of the failing heart before heart transplantation

C. Contraindications

1. Dissection of aortic or thoracic aneurysm
2. Incompetent aortic valve
3. Irreversible brain damage
4. Chronic end-stage heart disease
5. Severe femoral artery disease (an ascending aorta or aortic arch approach can be performed)

D. Complications

1. Dissection of the aorta
2. Thrombus formation
3. Impaired circulation distal to insertion site of the affected leg
4. Sepsis
5. Obstruction of blood flow to the left subclavian artery
6. Obstruction of blood flow to the renal arteries
7. Adverse effects caused by prolonged immobility

E. Patient care management

1. Observe for clinical signs of effectiveness
   a. Increased blood pressure
   b. Increased CO
   c. Improved mental alertness
   d. Increased urine output
   e. Warm, dry skin
   f. Palpable peripheral pulses
   g. Decreased chest pain
   h. Improved ischemic ECG changes
2. Assess and document continuous ECG rhythm, vital signs, mental status, heart and lung sounds, urine output, and any signs or symptoms indicating changes in these parameters
3. Monitor for and treat arrhythmias early because irregularity in the cardiac rhythm decreases IABP effectiveness
4. Monitor circulation in the affected leg by checking pulses, color, sensation, mobility, and temperature, and promptly report any changes
5. Keep the affected leg straight and logroll patient when turning

6. Keep head of the bed elevated 30 degrees or less to prevent upward migration of catheter
7. Assess for indications of catheter migration
   a. Decreased left radial pulse
   b. Sudden decrease in urine output
   c. Flank pain
   d. Dizziness or sudden change in level of consciousness
8. Monitor for IABP malfunction (persons caring for a patient with an IABP should receive formal training)
9. Monitor for adverse effects of anticoagulation
   a. Abnormal prothrombin time, partial thromboplastin time, or platelet count
   b. Positive stool guaiac test
   c. Positive nasogastric tube aspirate guaiac test
   d. Hematuria
   e. Oozing of blood from any orifices or the insertion site
10. Refer to patient care measures related to the specific condition for which IABP was implemented

♦ V. Ventricular assist device (VAD)

A. General information
1. The VAD is a mechanical heart-assist device that provides total support to the heart and circulation in patients who are unresponsive to drug therapy or IABP
2. It may be used to support the left ventricle (LVAD), the right ventricle (RVAD), or both ventricles (BIVAD)
3. Most VADs are used in conjunction with the IABP
4. Insertion of a VAD is more easily performed when the patient's chest is open, as with surgery
5. Blood is diverted from the heart and routed to the pump and is returned to the pulmonary artery (with RVAD) or aorta (with LVAD)
6. The VAD pump can generate a CO up to 10 liters/minute, which is adjusted by the operator of the pump, depending on the patient's needs
7. As the patient's condition improves, the patient is gradually weaned from the VAD; weaning from a BIVAD may be biphasic because each ventricle may recover at a different time
8. The goal is to provide sufficient CO that supports adequate tissue perfusion while allowing the heart to rest and recover from the insult

B. Uses
1. Cardiogenic shock
2. Postcardiac surgery in patients with low CO
3. Cardiomyopathy awaiting heart transplantation

C. Contraindications
  1. Prolonged cardiac arrest with central nervous system damage
  2. Irreversible myocardial damage, which may prevent weaning from the VAD
  3. Chronic liver disease
  4. Sepsis
  5. Severe renal failure

D. Complications
  1. Coagulopathies
  2. Surgery-related bleeding
  3. Embolization
  4. Sepsis
  5. Right ventricular failure (with LVAD only)
  6. Acute renal failure
  7. Neurologic deficits, such as transient ischemic attack and cerebrovascular accident

E. Patient care management
  1. Observe for clinical signs of VAD effectiveness
     a. Increased blood pressure
     b. Increased CO
     c. Improved mental alertness
     d. Increased urine output
     e. Warm, dry skin
     f. Palpable peripheral pulses
     g. Improved hemodynamic parameters (CO is accurate only with LVAD, not with RVAD)
  2. Assess and document continuous ECG rhythm, vital signs, level of consciousness, heart and lung sounds, urine output, and any signs or symptoms indicating changes in these parameters
  3. Maintain I.V. fluids as indicated to ensure that left atrial pressure is at least 10 mm Hg to prevent vacuum effect with LVAD
  4. Monitor for VAD malfunction (persons caring for a patient with a VAD should receive formal training)
  5. Monitor for complications associated with use of VAD
  6. Anticipate weaning from the VAD when patient's ventricle can maintain sufficient CO while temporarily off VAD (mean arterial pressure greater than 60 mm Hg, cardiac index greater than 2 liters/minute/m^2, right atrial and left atrial pressures less than 25 mm Hg)
  7. Refer to patient care measures related to the specific condition for which VAD was implemented

Points to remember

- Alternative management therapies are used to help patients with electrical or mechanical cardiac dysfunction.
- Cardiac pacing provides an extrinsic electrical impulse to initiate depolarization of the myocardium.
- The ICD analyzes a patient's cardiac rhythm and delivers an internal electrical charge when an arrhythmia is detected.
- The IABP is a counterpulsation device that assists the failing heart by decreasing myocardial oxygen demand.
- The patient care management goal for a patient with an IABP or a VAD is to provide CO that supports adequate tissue perfusion while allowing the heart to rest and recover from the insult.

Study questions

To evaluate your understanding of this chapter, answer the following questions in the space provided; then compare your responses with the correct answers in Appendix B, pages 282 and 283.

1. Which three routes are commonly used for insertion of a temporary pacemaker? ______________________________

____

____

2. What intervention should the nurse implement if a patient with a temporary pacemaker experiences cardiac arrest?______________________________

____

____

3. How does the ICD correct lethal ventricular arrhythmias?______________________________

____

____

4. What benefits are derived from the IABP's appropriately timed inflation and deflation of the balloon? ____________________

____

____

5. Which signs and symptoms of IABP catheter migration should the nurse watch for? ____________________

____

____

6. What clinical signs of VAD effectiveness should the nurse watch for? ______

____

____

CRITICAL THINKING AND APPLICATION EXERCISES

1. Observe a pacemaker placement. Prepare an oral presentation for your fellow students, describing the procedure and patient care measures before, during, and after the procedure.
2. Develop a chart comparing the commonly used alternative management therapies in cardiac care, including their uses, complications, and patient care management.
3. Talk to two patients who have had an ICD. Ask them for their opinion of it, and inquire whether their quality of life has changed.
4. Observe a patient with an IABP in place, and note the patient management activities that were performed while you observed. Report your findings to your classmates.

CHAPTER

13

Cardiovascular Disorders

Learning objectives

After studying this chapter, you should be able to:

- Describe the general principles of cardiovascular function.
- Identify the possible causes for each type of alteration in cardiovascular function.
- Discuss common assessment and diagnostic test findings for the patient with a specific alteration in cardiovascular function.
- Describe care management for the patient with a specific alteration in cardiovascular function.

Chapter overview

Cardiovascular disease is the leading cause of death in both men and women in the United States. Caring for the patient with a cardiovascular disorder in an emergency or critical care area requires a sound understanding of cardiovascular anatomy, physiology, and hemodynamic function. Various causes contribute to each type of alteration in cardiovascular function. Common assessment and diagnostic test findings are used to determine the type and extent of dysfunction. In general, patient care management is aimed at decreasing cardiac workload and increasing blood supply, thereby enhancing tissue perfusion.

♦ I. Introduction

A. Functions of the heart
   1. Pumps blood to the tissues
   2. Supplies oxygen and removes carbon dioxide and other metabolic waste products

B. Risk factors
   1. RISK FACTORS associated with increased risk of developing cardiovascular disease are classified as nonmodifiable, modifiable, and contributing
   2. *Nonmodifiable* risk factors include age, sex, and race
      a. Age: cardiovascular disease increases with age
      b. Sex: men have a greater risk of developing cardiovascular disease than do women before menopause; rates of cardiovascular disease in women over age 65 exceed men's rates
      c. Race: nonwhites have a greater risk of developing cardiovascular disease than do whites
   3. *Modifiable* risk factors include cigarette smoking, hypertension, increased serum cholesterol levels, and diabetes
   4. *Contributing* risk factors include obesity, physical inactivity, type A personality, and stress
   5. Cardiovascular disease is the leading cause of death in the United States for both men and women

C. Potential nursing diagnoses for patients with cardiovascular disorders
   1. Pain
   2. Decreased CARDIAC OUTPUT (CO)
   3. Activity intolerance
   4. Anxiety
   5. Ineffective individual coping
   6. Ineffective family coping
   7. Altered nutrition: less than body requirements
   8. Risk for injury
   9. Self-care deficit

♦ II. Anatomy and physiology

A. Blood supply
   1. Blood supply to the heart is provided by the coronary arteries
      a. Right coronary artery
      b. Left main coronary artery with major branches of the left anterior descending and circumflex arteries
      c. Collateral arteries that connect two branches of a single coronary artery or branches of the right with branches of the left; normally present but greatly enlarged with hypoxia or chronic anemia

2. Much variation exists in the pattern of coronary artery and collateral branching

B. Cardiac cycle

1. The cardiac cycle consists of diastole and systole
2. *Diastole,* the filling phase, occurs as the ventricles receive blood from the atria to provide stroke volume (SV); the coronary arteries are perfused during this phase
3. *Systole,* the ejection phase, occurs when ventricular pressure exceeds aortic pressure; 90% of myocardial oxygen consumption ($M\overline{V}O_2$) occurs during isometric contraction

C. Myocardial oxygen supply

1. Myocardial oxygen supply is determined by coronary artery anatomy, diastolic pressure, diastolic time, and oxygen extraction based on hemoglobin and partial pressure of oxygen in arterial blood
2. $M\overline{V}O_2$, which must be in balance with blood supply to the heart, is determined by CO

D. Cardiac output (CO)

1. CO measures cardiac performance and is calculated by multiplying the heart rate (HR) times the SV: $CO = HR \times SV$
2. Cardiac index is calculated by dividing CO by the body surface area (obtained from a standard chart) to adjust for body size (see Chapter 8)

E. Stroke volume

1. SV consists of preload, afterload, and contractility
2. *Preload* is the ventricular filling pressure at the end of diastole; clinical indicators are central venous pressure (CVP) on the right side of the heart and pulmonary artery wedge pressure (PAWP) on the left; preload is related to STARLING'S LAW
3. *Afterload* is the amount of pressure the left ventricle must overcome during systole to open the semilunar valves and eject blood; clinical indicators are pulmonary vascular resistance on the right side of the heart and systemic vascular resistance (SVR) on the left
4. *Contractility* relates to changes in the force of contraction independent of changes in myocardial fiber length or preload; clinical indicators of contractility are stroke work index, left ventricular stroke work index, and right ventricular stroke work index

F. Compensatory mechanisms

1. The heart uses compensatory mechanisms to increase CO, including increasing the heart rate, thickening the ventricular wall, and increasing the ventricular chamber size
2. As compensatory mechanisms fail to maintain CO, decompensation occurs

3. The normal aging heart can provide a CO of 4 to 6 liters/minute under normal conditions but may have limited compensatory ability to provide increased CO demanded by physically or emotionally stressful situations

♦ III. Angina pectoris

A. General information
1. Angina pectoris causes chest pain or discomfort from insufficient myocardial oxygen supply
2. Angina may be classified as stable, unstable, or variant
3. *Stable angina* is characterized by a consistent pattern of cause, intensity, and duration; the pain is relieved with rest, nitroglycerin, or both
4. *Unstable angina* is characterized by a change in the quality, duration, severity, or frequency of pain or by a change in the activity level that triggers pain
5. *Prinzmetal's* (or *variant*) *angina* is an atypical pain caused by coronary artery vasospasm and often is unrelated to activity or other stress

B. Causes
1. Coronary thrombosis over high-grade lesion
2. Coronary artery vasospasm
3. Increased oxygen demands
4. Decreased coronary artery perfusion pressure
5. Decreased diastolic filling time
6. Anemia

C. Assessment findings
1. Pain or discomfort precipitated by physical exercise, stress, cold, heavy meals, or smoking
2. Pain relief within 5 minutes from rest, nitroglycerin, or both
3. Retrosternal chest pain that may radiate to the jaw or shoulders or down one or both arms
4. Descriptions of tightness, squeezing, burning, or smothering rather than pain
5. Expression of fear of impending doom
6. Elevated blood pressure as a response to pain
7. Decreased blood pressure if chest pain is caused by ischemia, which causes decreased CO

D. Diagnostic test findings
1. Electrocardiogram (ECG): depressed ST segment, with or without T-wave inversion; elevated ST segment in Prinzmetal's angina dur-

ing an episode of chest pain; absence of ECG abnormality does not rule out disease

2. Stress testing: coronary artery disease (CAD)
3. Cardiac catheterization: atherosclerotic changes in coronary arteries
4. Complete blood count (CBC): anemia as the cause of chest pain

E. Patient care management

1. Goals
   a. Relieve acute pain
   b. Reduce cardiac workload
2. Strategies
   a. Administer oxygen to relieve ischemia at a flow rate based on institutional policy and the patient's condition
   b. Assess and document continuous ECG rhythm, vital signs, mental status, and heart and lung sounds
   c. Assess and document pain characteristics: location, duration, intensity (have patient grade pain on a scale from 1 to 10), precipitating factors, relief measures, and symptoms that indicate changes in these parameters
   d. Assess vital signs with complaints of chest pain, and compare with baseline
   e. Begin I.V. nitroglycerin titrated until acute pain is relieved; check blood pressure every 15 minutes or according to institutional policy; maintain systolic blood pressure greater than 90 mm Hg or according to institutional protocol; document the patient's response to therapy
   f. Administer I.V. morphine in small doses to relieve pain and decrease preload
   g. Give sublingual, oral, or topical nitroglycerin prophylactically for chronic pain
   h. Consider calcium channel blockers with Prinzmetal's angina to block the influx of calcium into the cell; calcium channel blockers produce vasodilation of coronary and peripheral arteries
   i. Use beta-adrenergic blockers to decrease myocardial oxygen demand by decreasing contractility, heart rate, and blood pressure
   j. Notify the doctor and obtain a 12-lead ECG at the onset of recurring chest pain
   k. Maintain activity restrictions based on the patient's activity tolerance to reduce myocardial oxygen demands
   l. Begin the patient on a low-cholesterol, low-sodium diet to alleviate the modifiable risk factors
   m. Consider percutaneous transluminal coronary angioplasty (PTCA) to improve blood flow through the stenotic coronary arteries

n. Remember that a coronary artery bypass graft (CABG) may be indicated when medical treatment has been unsuccessful, based on the patient's symptoms and the cardiac catheterization report
o. Provide patient education, and ensure that the patient can recognize signs and symptoms necessitating medical attention (unrelieved chest pain after taking three nitroglycerin tablets sublingually 5 minutes apart)
p. Work with the patient and family to identify the patient's risk factors and necessary lifestyle modifications
q. Refer the family to appropriate sources for cardiopulmonary resuscitation (CPR) training
r. Ensure that the family can activate the emergency medical system if any problems occur at home

♦ IV. Acute myocardial infarction (MI)

A. General information
1. MI causes the death of myocardial tissue from inadequate blood supply to the myocardium
2. MIs are classified according to the layer of myocardial tissue involved or the location of damage to the left ventricle
3. A *non–Q-wave* infarction, or *subendocardial* MI, is limited to the inner half of the ventricular muscle; a *Q-wave* infarction, or *transmural* MI, involves the entire thickness of the myocardium
4. An anterior MI usually involves occlusion of the left anterior descending (LAD) coronary artery; the ECG changes are seen in leads V_2 through V_4
5. An inferior or diaphragmatic MI usually involves occlusion of the right coronary artery; ECG changes are seen in leads II, III, and aV_F
6. A posterior MI involves occlusion of the right coronary artery or circumflex branch of the left coronary artery and, usually, the lateral or inferior wall of the left ventricle; reciprocal changes are seen in ECG leads V_1 and V_2 (the standard 12-lead ECG does not directly record electrical activity on the posterior surface so only reciprocal changes are seen)
7. A lateral MI is relatively rare, with damage confined to the lateral wall, although it may occur in combination with an anterior MI; ECG changes are seen in leads I, aV_F, V_5, and V_6
8. A septal MI involves occlusion of the LAD artery and involves the septum, which separates the left and right ventricles; ECG changes are seen in leads V_1 and V_2

9. Right ventricular (RV) infarction occurs when occlusion of the right coronary artery damages the right ventricle; it occurs most often with an inferior MI; a right-sided ECG can help with the diagnosis

CLINICAL ALERT

10. An anterior or lateral MI produces significantly higher mortality, more damage to the myocardium, more conduction disturbances, and increased occurrences of congestive heart failure (CHF) and cardiogenic shock than does an inferior or a posterior MI

B. Causes
1. Occlusion of coronary artery blood flow from coronary thrombus over a high-grade lesion
2. Coronary artery vasospasm
3. Increased oxygen demands
4. Decreased coronary artery perfusion pressure

C. Assessment findings
1. Substernal crushing chest pain that may radiate to the jaw, shoulders, or back or down one or both arms or may be asymptomatic
2. Pain unrelieved by rest, position, or nitroglycerin and lasting longer than 30 minutes
3. Dyspnea
4. Hypoxemia
5. Diaphoresis
6. Nausea or vomiting
7. Anxiety
8. Decreased blood pressure
9. Increased temperature

CLINICAL ALERT

D. Diagnostic test findings
1. Serum creatine kinase (CK-MB): CK-MB isoenzyme elevation greater than established institutional criterion that begins 4 to 8 hours after infarction, peaks at 24 hours, and lasts for 72 hours after infarction
2. Serum lactate dehydrogenase (LDH): LDH_1 level greater than LDH_2 level; this isoenzyme pattern of elevation develops 12 to 24 hours after infarction, peaks at 36 to 72 hours, and returns to normal within 10 days after the infarction
3. ECG: changes in leads over area of infarct: ST-segment elevation (indicating injury to myocardial tissue), ST-segment depression (in leads that view the opposite wall), T-wave flattening and inversion (indicating ischemia of the myocardial tissue), and Q-wave abnormalities (representing tissue death), which are clinically significant if the Q wave is greater than one-third of the total QRS height or wider than 0.04 second

4. Chest X-ray: cardiac enlargement and signs of left ventricular (LV) failure (pulmonary congestion); may also be normal
5. Echocardiogram: abnormalities of LV wall motion and valve competency
6. Hemodynamic monitoring: increased pulmonary artery pressure (PAP), increased PAWP, decreased CO, and increased SVR, depending on extent of the MI

E. Patient care management
   1. Goals
      a. Relieve acute pain
      b. Reduce cardiac workload
      c. Prevent and treat arrhythmias
      d. Manage fluid imbalances
      e. Limit infarct size by reperfusion
   2. Strategies
      a. Administer oxygen to relieve ischemia at a flow rate based on institutional policy and the patient's condition
      b. Assess and document characteristics of pain: location, duration, intensity
         (1) Have patient grade pain on a scale from 1 to 10
         (2) Note precipitating factors, relief measures, and associated symptoms

CLINICAL ALERT

         (3) Be aware that most of what the textbooks say about the "typical" symptoms of an MI was written about men and the findings have been applied to women; in fact, women present with different symptoms, including less crushing substernal chest pain, that are quite "typical" for them but no less concerning
      c. Assess and document continuous ECG rhythm, vital signs, mental status, heart and lung sounds, urine output, and any signs or symptoms indicating changes in these parameters
         (1) Monitor cardiac enzyme levels
         (2) Anticipate use of new diagnostic tests, including myoglobin and cardiac troponin
      d. Assess vital signs with symptoms of chest pain, and compare with baseline
      e. Begin I.V. nitroglycerin titrated until acute pain is relieved; check blood pressure every 15 minutes or according to institutional policy; maintain systolic blood pressure greater than 90 mm Hg or according to institutional protocol; document the patient's response to therapy

CLINICAL ALERT

f. Administer I.V. morphine in small doses to relieve pain, to reduce anxiety, and to decrease preload and $M\bar{V}O_2$
g. Know that prophylactic use of lidocaine has been shown in some studies to increase mortality during the hospital phase of a monitored, uncomplicated MI
h. Administer thrombolytic therapy with tissue plasminogen activator or streptokinase within the first few hours to lyse the clot after any chest pain suggesting an infarction
i. Keep in mind that the doctor may order anticoagulants to prevent clot formation
j. Keep in mind that beta blockers may also be ordered to decrease heart rate and contractility, helping balance supply and demand; avoid if patient is bradycardic, receiving thrombolytics, or having emergent PTCA
k. If a pulmonary artery catheter is in place, assess and document PAP, PAWP, CO, and SVR, as ordered
l. Run a 12-lead ECG when pain occurs and then daily for 3 days to evaluate any evolutionary changes associated with MI
m. Monitor serum potassium levels, and report levels outside normal limits; potassium levels should be kept higher than 4 mEq/liter to reduce the risk of arrhythmias
n. Enforce activity restrictions to decrease oxygen requirements
o. Maintain accurate intake and output records and daily weights to assess fluid status
p. Begin the patient on a low-cholesterol, low-sodium diet to alter modifiable risk factors
q. Consider PTCA to improve blood flow through the stenotic coronary arteries
r. Remember that a CABG may be indicated when medical treatment has been unsuccessful, based on the patient's symptoms and the cardiac catheterization report
s. Provide patient education (for specific teaching tips, see *Patient recovering from an MI*, page 120)

♦ V. Congestive heart failure

A. General information
1. CHF results from the heart's inability to maintain sufficient output to meet the body's metabolic demands

CLINICAL ALERT

2. Although CHF classically is associated with a defect in systolic function (systolic heart failure), patients may present in diastolic heart failure with an impaired ability of the ventricle to accept blood; patient care management in this group differs

TEACHING TIPS

Patient recovering from an MI

Be sure to include the following topics in your teaching plan for a patient recovering from a myocardial infarction (MI).

- Explanation of MI and what it means
- Signs and symptoms necessitating medical attention, such as unrelieved chest pain after taking three nitroglycerin tablets sublingually 5 minutes apart
- Guidelines for resuming sexual activity after discharge
- Risk factors
- Necessary lifestyle modifications, such as smoking cessation and stress management
- Dietary modifications and restrictions
- Medication regimen, including dosage, scheduling, and adverse effects
- Signs and symptoms of complications
- Cardiopulmonary resuscitation training for family members
- Emergency medical service activation at home if problems occur
- Medical follow-up

3. Most commonly, CHF (from systolic failure) is classified as LV and RV failure
4. *LV failure* occurs when the left ventricle cannot pump blood efficiently from the lungs to the systemic circulation
5. Pressure increases in the lungs from the accumulation of blood; as this pressure exceeds the pulmonary capillary oncotic pressure, fluid leaks into the pulmonary interstitial space, causing pulmonary edema
6. LV failure commonly occurs suddenly, making the compensatory mechanisms ineffective
7. *RV failure* occurs when the right ventricle cannot pump blood efficiently from venous return into the pulmonary system
8. As the pressure backs up in the systemic circulation, body organs become congested with venous blood
9. The most common characteristic of heart failure is low CO; in certain situations (thyrotoxicosis, pregnancy, anemia, beriberi, Paget's disease), high CO also may lead to heart failure secondary to unusually high metabolic demands that exceed the ability of an otherwise healthy heart

B. Causes: LV failure

1. CAD
2. Hypertension
3. Cigarette smoking
4. Obesity
5. Increased stress

6. Sedentary lifestyle
7. Diabetes

C. Causes: RV failure
1. Mitral valve stenosis
2. Acute RV infarctions
3. Pulmonary embolus
4. Chronic obstructive pulmonary disease
5. LV failure

D. Assessment findings: LV failure
1. Moist cough with frothy sputum
2. Dyspnea
3. Crackles
4. S_3 or S_4 HEART SOUNDS
5. Anxiety
6. Diaphoresis
7. Decreased blood pressure
8. Tachycardia
9. Arrhythmias
10. PULSUS ALTERNANS

E. Assessment findings: RV failure
1. Fluid retention
2. Jugular vein distention
3. Peripheral edema
4. Decreased urine output
5. Hepatojugular reflux
6. Bounding pulses
7. Ascites

F. Diagnostic test findings
1. Chest X-ray: pulmonary congestion or CARDIOMEGALY
2. Arterial blood gas analysis: hypoxemia or respiratory alkalosis
3. ECG: LV and RV hypertrophy or arrhythmias
4. Serum electrolyte studies: hyponatremia (dilutional) or hypokalemia
5. CBC: decreased hemoglobin and hematocrit levels (dilutional or anemic)
6. Hemodynamic monitoring: LV failure — increased PAP, PAWP, CVP, or right atrial pressure (RAP); decreased CO, RV failure — increased PAP, CVP, or RAP; normal PAWP

G. Patient care management
1. Goals
   a. Treat underlying or precipitating factors
   b. Reduce cardiac workload

2. Strategies
   a. Provide oxygen to relieve ischemia at a flow rate based on institutional policy and the patient's condition
   b. Assess and document continuous ECG rhythm, vital signs, mental status, heart and lung sounds, urine output, and signs or symptoms indicating changes in these parameters
   c. Maintain activity restrictions based on the patient's activity tolerance to reduce myocardial oxygen demands
   d. Administer I.V. morphine in small doses to decrease venous return, preload, $M\bar{V}O_2$, pain, and anxiety
   e. Begin diuretics to decrease preload and blood volume
   f. Start digitalis to increase contractility and decrease heart rate
   g. Consider vasopressors to increase contractility and support blood pressure
   h. Use nitrates to decrease preload and pulmonary and cardiac congestion
   i. Use afterload-reducing agents to decrease SVR and aid ventricular ejection
   j. If a pulmonary artery catheter is in place, assess and document PAP, PAWP, CO, and SVR, as ordered
   k. Provide patient education, and ensure that the patient can recognize signs and symptoms necessitating medical attention (for example, increased shortness of breath, weight gain, decreased activity tolerance, or change in pulse rate or rhythm) and understands dietary restrictions
   l. Refer the family to appropriate sources for CPR training
   m. Ensure that the family can activate the emergency medical system if any problems occur at home

♦ VI. Cardiomyopathy

A. General information
   1. Cardiomyopathy is a subacute or chronic disorder involving an abnormality of the ventricular muscle that causes heart failure
   2. Classification is made by physiologic, pathological, and clinical signs; cardiomyopathy is classified as dilated, hypertrophic, or restrictive
   3. *Dilated cardiomyopathy* demonstrates enlarged ventricular cavity, little or no hypertrophy of muscle wall, and decreased systolic ejection fraction
   4. *Hypertrophic cardiomyopathy* produces an abnormally stiff left ventricle that limits ventricular filling; thickening of the septum impairs blood outflow from the ventricle and is called idiopathic hypertrophic subaortic stenosis

5. *Restrictive cardiomyopathy* leads to impaired ventricular stretch and diastolic filling
6. Regardless of the category, the course of cardiomyopathy is progressive, leading to impaired LV ejection, blood stasis in the ventricle and eventually the atrium, increased preload and afterload, and CHF
7. Cardiomyopathy may also be classified according to cause as primary or secondary
   a. *Primary cardiomyopathy* results from an unknown cause
   b. *Secondary cardiomyopathy* results from a systemic disorder
8. When heart failure from cardiomyopathy progresses to a point beyond medical responsiveness, the only hope for the patient's survival is a heart transplant

B. Causes
1. Idiopathic origin
2. Excessive alcohol intake
3. Infections
4. Hypertension
5. Metabolic diseases
6. Toxic responses
7. Immune diseases
8. Neoplastic heart disease

C. Assessment findings
1. Dyspnea on exertion
2. Hypotension
3. Ischemic chest pain
4. S_3 or S_4 heart sounds
5. Crackles
6. Murmurs
7. Paroxysmal nocturnal dyspnea
8. Easy fatigability
9. Cough

D. Diagnostic test findings: diagnosis is commonly made by ruling out other diseases
1. Chest X-ray: pulmonary congestion or cardiomegaly
2. ECG: atrial fibrillation, tachycardia, ventricular ectopy, or left axis deviation
3. Echocardiogram: abnormalities of LV wall motion, dilation of cardiac chambers, and valve competency
4. Cardiac catheterization: rules out coronary disease as causative factor

E. Patient care management
1. Goal: to reestablish and maintain hemodynamic stability

2. Strategies
   a. Administer oxygen to relieve ischemia at a flow rate based on institutional policy and the patient's condition
   b. Enforce activity restrictions to reduce myocardial oxygen demands
   c. Use vasodilators to decrease preload and afterload and to improve CO
   d. Use diuretics to reduce preload and pulmonary congestion
   e. Consider inotropic agents to increase myocardial contractility
   f. Begin calcium channel blockers to decrease cardiac workload through vasodilation
   g. Consider beta blockers for hypertrophic cardiomyopathy to reduce outflow obstruction during exercise
   h. Consider anticoagulants to prevent clot formation associated with atrial fibrillation
   i. If a pulmonary artery catheter is in place, assess and document PAP, PAWP, CO, and SVR, as ordered
   j. Provide patient education, and ensure that the patient can recognize signs and symptoms necessitating medical attention (for example, increased shortness of breath, weight gain, decreased activity tolerance, or change in pulse rate or rhythm) and understands that the disease is chronic and requires ongoing management and treatment
   k. Work with the patient to devise a plan for risk factor modification (such as alcohol abstinence and diet restrictions)

♦ VII. Cardiac tamponade

A. General information
1. Cardiac tamponade is a sudden accumulation of blood or fluid within the pericardial space, causing heart compression and interfering with cardiac filling and ejection
2. The pericardial sac normally contains 10 to 30 ml of fluid that protects the myocardium; it has limited stretching ability
3. Clinical manifestations depend on the rate of fluid accumulation
4. A sudden addition of 50 to 100 ml of fluid can cause a rise in intrapericardial pressure
5. As intrapericardial pressure exceeds CVP, the heart chambers and the coronary arteries are compressed
6. When cardiac filling and ejection are impaired, CO decreases and tissue perfusion is compromised
7. Circulatory collapse can occur if acute cardiac tamponade is not corrected immediately

B. Causes
1. Blunt or penetrating trauma to chest
2. Complications from central line placement, cardiac catheterization, pacemaker insertion, or angiography
3. MI
4. Acute pericarditis
5. Malignant metastases to the pericardium
6. Kidney or liver failure

C. Assessment findings: depend on the rate of fluid accumulation
1. Hypotension
2. Tachycardia
3. Cold, clammy skin
4. Dyspnea
5. Precordial pain
6. Muffled heart sounds
7. Jugular vein distention
8. Pulsus paradoxus
9. Anxiety

D. Diagnostic test findings
1. ECG: ST-segment elevation or nonspecific ST and T-wave changes
2. Chest X-ray: normal or enlarged cardiac silhouette or widened mediastinum
3. Echocardiogram: right-to-left shift of intraventricular septum with inspiration; echo-free space in front of RV wall and behind LV wall

E. Patient care management
1. Goal: to reestablish and maintain hemodynamic stability
2. Strategies
   a. Anticipate performance of pericardiocentesis to drain pericardial space of excess fluid
   b. Assess and document continuous ECG rhythm, vital signs, mental status, heart and lung sounds, urine output, and any signs or symptoms indicating changes in these parameters
   c. Consider pericardiostomy to drain pericardial space
   d. Initiate I.V. volume therapy with fluids and volume expanders through a large-bore peripheral I.V. line to increase diastolic filling pressure for improved CO
   e. Administer oxygen to correct hypoxia at a flow rate based on institutional policy and the patient's condition
   f. Consider inotropic agents to increase contractility
   g. Begin resuscitative measures, if necessary

VIII. Hypertensive crisis

A. General information
   1. Hypertensive crisis is a severe, fixed elevation of the resting arterial pressure, which may produce vascular necrosis as diastolic pressure exceeds 140 mm Hg
   2. The speed of increase in recorded pressure may be more destructive than the actual blood pressure
   3. The mortality associated with hypertensive crisis that is untreated for 1 year is 75%

B. Causes
   1. Inadequately treated or untreated essential hypertension
   2. Poor compliance with treatment plan
   3. Renal disease

C. Assessment findings
   1. Diastolic blood pressure above 140 mm Hg
   2. Throbbing headache
   3. Renal impairment
   4. Vision loss
   5. Confusion
   6. Signs of heart failure (moist cough with frothy sputum, dyspnea, crackles, or S_3 or S_4 heart sounds)

D. Diagnostic test findings
   1. Blood pressure measurements: severely elevated
   2. Funduscopic eye examination: retinal changes (hemorrhages, exudates, narrowed arterioles, and papilledema)
   3. ECG: LV hypertrophy
   4. Chest X-ray: cardiomegaly and pulmonary congestion if heart failure is present

E. Patient care management
   1. Goals
      a. Reduce blood pressure rapidly
      b. Prevent further hypertensive episodes
   2. Strategies

CLINICAL ALERT

      a. Administer I.V. nitroprusside (drug of choice) to cause immediate vasodilation; mix the drug only in dextrose 5% in water
         (1) Keep the bag protected from light
         (2) Assess for possible thiocyanate toxicity (nausea, tinnitus, or fatigue)
         (3) Measure serum thiocyanate levels every 72 hours

CLINICAL ALERT

b. Monitor blood pressure every 5 minutes or according to institutional policy during titration of medications
c. Use direct arterial pressure monitoring or automatic blood pressure cuff monitoring to evaluate blood pressure accurately and continuously and to prevent hypotension with drug titration
d. Assess and document continuous ECG rhythm, mental status, heart and lung sounds, urine output, and any signs or symptoms indicating changes in these parameters
e. Evaluate changes in visual acuity by assessing the patient's ability to recognize objects and people
f. Consider I.V. diazoxide instead of nitroprusside to vasodilate arterial smooth muscle
g. Administer I.V. labetalol hydrochloride instead of nitroprusside to block alpha and beta sympathetic response
h. Begin oral antihypertensive therapy after acute episode is controlled so that the patient can be weaned off I.V. drugs
i. Maintain bed rest to minimize oxygen requirements

CLINICAL ALERT

j. Be aware that a patient admitted to the emergency or intensive care area may have antihypertensive therapy inadvertently interrupted, which may cause a rebound elevation of blood pressure
k. Provide patient education, and ensure that the patient understands the importance of continuing treatment even when feeling well, can take accurate blood pressure readings and keep daily records as directed, and recognizes the importance of complying with prescribed activity after blood pressure is controlled
l. Work with the patient to devise a plan for risk factor modification (for example, smoking cessation, stress management, and diet restrictions)

POINTS TO REMEMBER

- The main compensatory mechanisms the heart uses to maintain CO are increasing the heart rate, thickening the ventricular wall, and increasing the chamber size of the ventricle.
- Cardiovascular disease remains the leading cause of death in the United States.
- The diagnosis of MI is based on patient history, signs and symptoms, cardiac enzyme levels, and ECG changes.
- Evaluation of the cardiovascular disease risk factors is an essential part of cardiovascular assessment.

STUDY QUESTIONS

To evaluate your understanding of this chapter, answer the following questions in the space provided; then compare your responses with the correct answers in Appendix B, pages 283 and 284.

1. Which of the cardiovascular risk factors are classed as modifiable or contributing? ____

2. During which phase of the cardiac cycle does coronary artery perfusion occur? ____

3. What differences in chest pain pattern are noted in the patient with angina versus MI? ____

4. What key diagnostic tests are used to diagnose an acute MI? ____________

5. What are common assessment findings in left-sided heart failure? ________

6. Which classifications of medication are used to relieve and maintain hemodynamic stability in a patient with cardiomyopathy? ______________

7. What patient care interventions are used to treat cardiac tamponade? _____

8. What is the drug of choice for treatment of hypertensive crisis? ________
____
____

CRITICAL THINKING AND APPLICATION EXERCISES

1. Develop a chart comparing the major drug classifications used for treating an MI.
2. Obtain a 3-day food history from a fellow student. Evaluate the information for possible cardiovascular risk factors, and identify ways to modify them.
3. List two strategies that can be used to enhance compliance in a patient with hypertension.
4. Develop a chart that shows the differences among dilated, hypertrophic, and restrictive cardiomyopathy in relation to cause, pathophysiology, and patient care management.
5. Follow a patient with a cardiovascular disorder from admission through discharge. Develop a plan of care, including any need for follow-up and home care.

CHAPTER

14

Respiratory Disorders

Learning objectives

After studying this chapter, you should be able to:

- Describe the general principles of respiratory system function.
- Identify possible causes for each type of alteration in respiratory function.
- Discuss common assessment and diagnostic test findings for the patient with a specific respiratory disorder.
- Describe care management for the patient with a specific alteration in respiratory function.

Chapter overview

Caring for the patient with a respiratory disorder requires an understanding of respiratory anatomy and physiology. A thorough assessment is essential to planning and implementing care. The assessment includes a history, identification of causes and risk factors, examination for signs and symptoms, and diagnostic test findings. Nursing diagnoses focus primarily on impaired gas exchange, ineffective airway clearance, anxiety, activity intolerance, and risk for infection. The major goals of patient care management are to maintain a patent airway, support ventilation, and maintain adequate arterial oxygenation to meet tissue demands.

♦ I. Introduction

A. Function
1. The primary function of the respiratory system is to provide oxygen for all metabolic processes and to remove carbon dioxide (CO_2)
2. Most patients in critical care units and many who present to emergency departments have some degree of respiratory dysfunction
   a. A critically ill patient may not have the reserve or the normal compensatory mechanisms to prevent pulmonary complications
   b. A critically ill patient may not be able to cough

B. Risk factors
1. History of airway obstruction from aspiration, inflammation, laryngitis, chronic lung disease, pulmonary edema, or near drowning
2. Thoracic restriction from trauma, flail chest, ruptured diaphragm, surgery, obesity, ascites, or arthritis involving the vertebral column
3. History of neuromuscular deficits, such as central nervous system (CNS) depression from drugs or trauma, coma, polio, multiple sclerosis, or Guillain-Barré syndrome
4. History of parenchymal disease caused by trauma to the lung tissue from contusion, tumors, or acute respiratory distress syndrome (ARDS, or shock lung)
5. Disturbance of pulmonary perfusion from emboli or pulmonary hypertension

C. Major management goal for a patient with a respiratory disorder: maintenance of a patent airway

D. Possible nursing diagnoses for a patient with a respiratory disorder
1. Impaired gas exchange
2. Ineffective airway clearance
3. Activity intolerance
4. Anxiety
5. Risk for infection

♦ II. Anatomy and physiology

A. Gas exchange
1. Adequate gas exchange is essential for proper functioning of all body systems
2. Normal stimulus for respiration is an increase in partial pressures of CO_2 in arterial blood ($Paco_2$)
3. In chronic lung disease, the stimulus for respiration when $Paco_2$ is consistently elevated is a decrease in partial pressures of oxygen (Pao_2)

B. Regulation
1. Respirations are regulated by mechanical and chemical factors
2. They are influenced by lung distensibility (compliance) and by the size of airways and the resistance to the flow they impart

C. Secondary functions
1. Regulation of acid-base balance through the expiration or retention of CO_2
2. Expression of emotion, such as sighing or laughing
3. Regulation of water balance and temperature control through water evaporation during respirations

♦ III. Respiratory acidosis

A. General information
1. RESPIRATORY ACIDOSIS is not a disease but an acid-base imbalance that results from any condition that interferes with pulmonary gas exchange and causes retention of CO_2 (hypoventilation)
2. The excess CO_2 then combines with water to form carbonic acid, increasing the carbonic acid level in the blood
3. Respiratory acidosis is classified as uncompensated or compensated
   a. *Uncompensated respiratory acidosis* is characterized by a sudden onset, with high $Paco_2$ levels and a sharp decrease in serum pH that occur before the renal system begins to compensate (usually takes hours to days)
   b. *Compensated respiratory acidosis* is characterized by the body's adaptation (COMPENSATION) to higher-than-normal CO_2 levels by the renal system, which allows retention of bicarbonate (HCO_3^-) to balance the elevated level of CO_2; produces a normal or near-normal Ph

B. Causes
1. Oversedation
2. Neuromuscular disorders
3. Trauma or surgery to the chest
4. Obstructive lung disease
5. Inappropriate mechanical ventilation
6. Any condition contributing to hypoventilation

C. Assessment findings: early signs and symptoms are related to CNS depression
1. Depressed rate and depth of respirations
2. Headache
3. Confusion
4. Lethargy
5. Arrhythmias
6. Dehydration

7. Slow, deep respiration or coma
8. Cyanosis
9. Elevated intracranial pressure (chronic)
10. Dilated conjunctival and facial blood vessels from hypercapnia (chronic)
11. Edema from right ventricular failure (chronic)

D. Diagnostic test findings
1. Chest X-ray: possible underlying pulmonary disease
2. Arterial blood gas (ABG) measurements: uncompensated, pH less than 7.35, Pa_{CO_2} greater than 45 mm Hg, HCO_3^- normal; compensated, pH normal, Pa_{CO_2} greater than 45 mm Hg, HCO_3^- greater than 26 mEq/liter, Pa_{O_2} less than 60 mm Hg (if hypoxia is a causative factor)
3. Electrocardiogram (ECG): arrhythmias present with acidosis, hypoxia, or electrolyte imbalances

E. Patient care management
1. Goals
   a. Support respiration
   b. Restore acid-base balance
2. Strategies
   a. Intubate and mechanically ventilate the patient if he or she cannot maintain breathing
   b. Administer oxygen therapy if hypoxia is present
      (1) Monitor Sa_{O_2} with pulse oximeter

CLINICAL ALERT

      (2) Use caution if hypoxia is a stimulus to breathe and the patient is not on mechanical ventilation because the ventilatory drive may be depressed and result in respiratory arrest
   c. Suction as necessary to remove secretions
   d. Administer bronchodilators to dilate smooth muscles of large airways
   e. Administer antibiotics appropriate for causative organism if infection is present
   f. Avoid use of narcotics and sedatives to
   g. Avoid use of HCO_3^- unless a base deficit exists
   h. Assess and document continuous ECG rhythm; vital signs; mental status; heart, lung, and bowel sounds; urine output; and any signs and symptoms indicating changes in these parameters
   i. Obtain ABG measurements and monitor for hypoxemia, hypercapnia, and acid-base imbalance
   j. Monitor laboratory results and report all abnormal values (serum potassium level may decrease as acidosis is reversed)
   k. Position the patient for comfort; elevate the head of the bed to facilitate gas exchange

l. Have the patient turn, cough, and deep-breathe to aid gas exchange and perfusion
m. Provide emotional support to decrease fear and anxiety
n. Teach the patient to recognize the signs and symptoms of the disease that require medical attention
o. Teach the patient techniques for improving lung function, such as deep or pursed-lip breathing

♦ IV. Respiratory alkalosis

A. General information

1. RESPIRATORY ALKALOSIS is not a disease but an acid-base imbalance that results from any condition that interferes with pulmonary gas exchange and causes excessive loss of CO_2 (hyperventilation)
2. Excessive loss of CO_2 causes a corresponding loss of carbonic acid in the blood
3. Respiratory alkalosis is classified as uncompensated or compensated
   a. *Uncompensated respiratory alkalosis* is characterized by sudden onset with low Pa_{CO_2} levels and a sharp increase in serum pH that occur before the renal system begins to compensate (usually takes hours to days)
   b. *Compensated respiratory alkalosis* is characterized by the body's adaptation to lower-than-normal CO_2 levels by the renal system, which allows excretion of HCO_3^- to balance the decrease in CO_2; produces a normal or near-normal pH

B. Causes

1. Anxiety
2. Hyperventilation
3. Pulmonary emboli
4. Pulmonary edema
5. Fever
6. Sepsis
7. Salicylate poisoning or overdose
8. Excessive mechanical ventilation
9. Pregnancy
10. Chronic hepatic insufficiency

C. Assessment findings: early signs and symptoms are related to excitability of the peripheral and central nervous systems; compensated respiratory alkalosis is usually asymptomatic

1. Increased rate and depth of respirations
2. Dizziness
3. Numbness or tingling in fingers and toes
4. Sweating
5. Muscle weakness

6. Tetany
7. Seizures
8. Syncope
9. Arrhythmias

D. Diagnostic test findings
1. Chest X-ray: possible underlying pulmonary disease
2. ABG measurements: uncompensated, pH greater than 7.45, $Paco_2$ less than 35 mm Hg, HCO_3^- normal; compensated, pH normal, $Paco_2$ less than 35 mm Hg, HCO_3^- less than 22 mEq/liter, Pao_2 less than 60 mm Hg, if hypoxia is a causative factor (for more information, see *Using ABGs to assess respiratory acid-base imbalances,* page 136)
3. ECG: arrhythmias with alkalosis, hypoxia, or electrolyte imbalance

E. Patient care management
1. Goals
a. Support respiration
b. Restore acid-base balance
2. Strategies
a. Use a rebreather mask or reservoir to increase the CO_2 level

CLINICAL ALERT

b. Administer oxygen therapy if hypoxia is present
c. Administer sedatives or analgesics if anxiety or pain is a causative factor
d. Consider changing the delivery mode of mechanical ventilation or parameter settings for tidal volume and rate
e. Provide emotional support to decrease fear and anxiety
f. Assess and document continuous ECG rhythm; vital signs; mental status; heart, lung, and bowel sounds; urine output; and any signs and symptoms indicating changes in these parameters
g. Obtain ABG measurements and monitor for hypoxemia and acid-base imbalances
h. Monitor laboratory results and report all abnormal values (serum potassium level may increase as alkalosis is reversed)
i. Teach the patient relaxation techniques to decrease anxiety

♦ V. Pneumonia

A. General information
1. Pneumonia is a bacterial, viral, or fungal infection that causes inflammation of the lung tissue
2. Pneumonia commonly impairs gas exchange
3. Pneumonia is classified according to cause (bacterial, viral, fungal, or protozoal), location (bronchopneumonia, lobular, or lobar), or type (primary, secondary, or aspiration)

DECISION TREE

Using ABGs to assess respiratory acid-base imbalances

To help determine if a patient is experiencing a respiratory acid-base imbalance, follow the decision tree steps below to interpret the patient's ABGs.

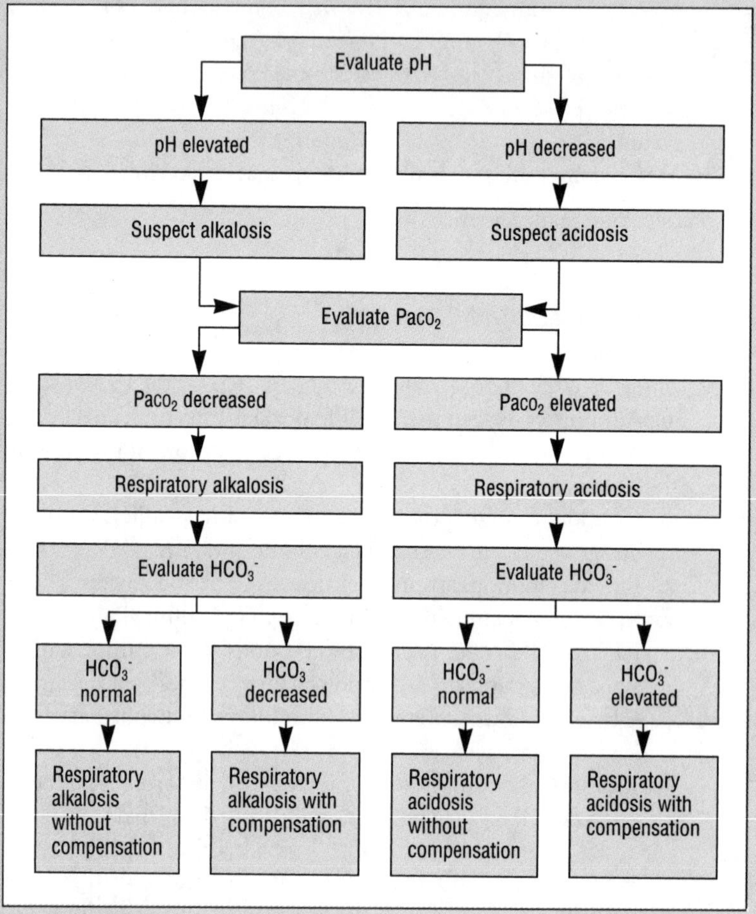

4. Twelve to fifteen percent of all patients in critical care areas contract pneumonia
5. Risk is increased in an elderly, immunocompromised, or chronically ill patient
6. Onset of signs and symptoms is influenced by age, extent of disease, and causative organism

B. Causes
1. Aspiration
2. Immunosuppression
3. Prolonged oxygen therapy
4. Immobility

C. Assessment findings
1. Productive or nonproductive cough (may be suppressed in a critically ill patient)
2. Mucoid, rusty, bloody, or purulent sputum
3. Fever
4. Chills
5. Pleuritic pain
6. Tachypnea
7. Tachycardia
8. Nasal flaring
9. Use of accessory muscles for breathing
10. Respiratory crackles, bronchial breath sounds

D. Diagnostic test findings
1. Chest X-ray: atelectasis, pleural effusion, consolidation, and inflammation
2. Sputum analysis for culture and sensitivity: identification of causative organism for effective antibiotic
3. White blood cell (WBC) count: elevated in bacterial infection and normal or decreased in viral or mycoplasmic infection
4. ABG measurements: hypoxemia and acid-base imbalances
5. Blood culture: bacteria in the blood

E. Patient care management
1. Goals
   a. Treat the infection
   b. Restore adequate ventilation for tissue perfusion
2. Strategies

CLINICAL ALERT

   a. Administer oxygen therapy if hypoxia is present
   b. Intubate and mechanically ventilate the patient if he or she cannot maintain breathing
   c. Suction as necessary to remove secretions
   d. Administer I.V. fluids for hydration and antibiotic therapy
   e. Administer antibiotics appropriate for the causative organism
   f. Administer antipyretics for fever, as necessary
   g. Administer analgesics for pleuritic pain
   h. Assess and document continuous ECG rhythm; vital signs; mental status; heart, lung, and bowel sounds; urine output; and any signs and symptoms indicating changes in these parameters

i. Monitor sputum production for color, viscosity, odor, and quantity
j. Schedule activities between periods of rest to conserve energy and decrease oxygen demand
k. Prevent transmission of infection by washing hands thoroughly and by wearing gloves when contact with blood or body fluids is likely
l. Observe infection-control and isolation procedures and precautions as defined by the Centers for Disease Control and Prevention and institutional policy
m. Teach the patient techniques for improving lung function, such as deep breathing, coughing, and spirometry exercises
n. Help the patient identify the need for therapeutic assistance to stop smoking, if necessary
o. Teach the patient the importance of balancing activity with rest to improve activity tolerance

♦ VI. Status asthmaticus

A. General information
1. Status asthmaticus is a severe, prolonged asthma attack that does not respond to traditional therapy of epinephrine and aminophylline
2. Onset may be rapid but usually is gradual, occurring over several days
3. Status asthmaticus is characterized by airway obstruction resulting from a spasm of the bronchial smooth muscle, mucosal edema, and the hypersecretion of mucus
4. Obstructed airways interfere with gas exchange and increase airway resistance
5. Severe elevation in intrathoracic pressures may interfere with venous return and cardiac output (CO), resulting in paradoxical pulses and blood pressure in which quality and pressures decrease with inspiration

B. Causes
1. Respiratory infections
2. Exposure to allergens, such as smoke and dust
3. Drug reaction
4. Failure to take prescribed asthma medications
5. Stress

C. Assessment findings
1. Extreme dyspnea with prolonged expiration
2. Nasal flaring
3. Use of accessory muscles

CLINICAL ALERT

4. Diminished breath sounds
5. Prolonged wheezing on expiration; wheezing may be absent if there is insufficient airflow through the airways or respiratory collapse
6. Cough; nonproductive or with thick, tenacious sputum
7. Tachypnea
8. Tachycardia; rapid, thready pulse with paradoxes
9. Chest tightness
10. Fatigue
11. Anxiety or fear

D. Diagnostic test findings
1. Chest X-ray: hyperinflation
2. ABG measurements: initially, severe hypoxemia, normal pH, and low $PaCO_2$ because of hyperventilation; followed by an elevation in $PaCO_2$ and a decrease in pH
3. Pulmonary function tests: decreased forced vital capacity and forced expiratory volume
4. Complete blood count: increased eosinophils (indicate allergic response if the patient is not taking steroids)
5. Sputum analysis for culture and sensitivity: identification of causative organism if infection is present

E. Patient care management
1. Goal: restore adequate ventilation for tissue perfusion
2. Strategies
   a. Administer humidified oxygen therapy to correct hypoxia
   b. Intubate and mechanically ventilate the patient if he or she cannot maintain breathing
   c. Suction as necessary to remove secretions
   d. Administer I.V. fluids for hydration and medication therapy
   e. Administer bronchodilators to dilate smooth muscles of large airways
   f. Administer corticosteroids to decrease inflammatory response
   g. Administer antibiotics appropriate for the causative organism, if infection is present
   h. Administer sedatives or tranquilizers for agitation, if necessary, to encourage the patient's cooperation with therapy, such as mechanical ventilation
   i. Assess and document continuous ECG rhythm; vital signs; mental status; heart, lung, and bowel sounds; urine output; and any signs and symptoms indicating changes in these parameters
   j. Obtain ABG measurements and monitor for hypoxemia and acid-base imbalance
   k. Monitor sputum production for color, viscosity, and quantity

l. Position the patient for comfort; elevate the head of the bed to facilitate respiration
m. Have the patient turn, cough, and deep-breathe to aid gas exchange and perfusion
n. Provide emotional support to decrease fear and anxiety
o. Help the patient and family to identify allergens or irritants that may precipitate an attack
p. Teach the patient how to monitor respiratory functioning by using forced expiratory flow, such as forced expiratory volume in 1 second or peak expiratory flow (for specific teaching tips, see *Patient with asthma*)
q. Develop emergency action plan for patient and family

♦ VII. Pulmonary embolism (PE)

A. General information
1. PE is a blockage of a pulmonary artery by foreign matter, such as a thrombus, fat, a tumor, tissue, air, amniotic fluid, or particulate matter, such as a catheter fragment
2. Substances released from the blockage cause constriction of the bronchial passages, decreasing lung volume and compliance
3. Hypoxemia arises from ventilation-perfusion ($\dot{V}/\dot{Q}$) mismatch
4. Alveolar collapse and atelectasis develop because the alveoli cannot produce enough SURFACTANT to maintain alveolar integrity; these factors increase pulmonary artery pressure (PAP) and intrapulmonary shunting
5. PE is one of the most common acute respiratory disorders in hospitalized patients
6. Approximately one-half of the PEs that cause death are undiagnosed
7. Onset of signs and symptoms usually is sudden and requires prompt detection and intervention

B. Causes
1. Stasis of the blood because of immobility
2. Deep-vein thrombosis
3. Clotting abnormalities
4. Atrial fibrillation
5. Myocardial infarction
6. Pelvic or abdominal surgery
7. Pregnancy or estrogen therapy
8. Trauma caused by long bone fractures (fat emboli)

C. Assessment findings
1. Sharp, sudden pleuritic chest pain
2. Dyspnea
3. Tachypnea with splinting

TEACHING TIPS
Patient with asthma

Be sure to include the following topics in your teaching plan for the asthmatic patient.

- Recording peak flow readings
- Maintaining an asthma symptom diary
- Correct use of metered-dose inhalers and bronchodilators
- Correct use of a peak flowmeter to determine the patient's best baseline flow rate and to monitor daily status
  – Green (safe) zone: 80% to 100% of best baseline value
  – Yellow (caution) zone: 50% to 80% of best baseline value, with coughing or wheezing that may prevent normal activity
  – Red (emergency) zone: less than 50% of best baseline value
- Identification of patterns in signs and symptoms to detect worsening airflow obstruction
- Avoidance of known irritants and allergens
- Allergen-proofing the home
- Medical follow-up and compliance with therapy

4. Restlessness and anxiety
5. Cough with possible HEMOPTYSIS
6. Tachycardia
7. Petechiae on anterior chest, neck, and axilla if the source is a fat embolus
8. Fever and diaphoresis
9. S_3 or S_4 heart sounds
10. Pleural friction rub

CLINICAL ALERT

11. Positive Homans' sign: absence of pain in the calf with dorsiflexion of the foot does not rule out a PE

D. Diagnostic test findings
1. Chest X-ray: may be normal
2. ABG measurements: hypoxemia and acid-base imbalances
3. ECG: right axis deviation; tall, peaked T waves; ST-segment changes; and T-wave inversion in leads V_1 through V_4
4. $\dot{V}/\dot{Q}$ scans: ventilation-perfusion mismatch (interruption of blood flow to affected lung area)
5. Pulmonary angiography (definitive test but invasive): location and extent of embolus
6. Hemodynamic monitoring: increased pulmonary vascular resistance evidenced by elevated PAP

E. Patient care management
   1. Goals
      a. Restore normal tissue perfusion
      b. Decrease risk of further obstruction
   2. Strategies
      a. Administer oxygen therapy to correct hypoxia
      b. Prepare the patient for pulmonary artery catheter placement to monitor fluid levels and evaluate therapy
      c. Assess and document central venous pressure (CVP), PAP, pulmonary artery wedge pressure (PAWP), CO, pulmonary vascular resistance (PVR), and systemic vascular resistance (SVR)
      d. Assess and document continuous ECG rhythm; vital signs; mental status; heart, lung, and bowel sounds; urine output; and any signs and symptoms indicating changes in these parameters
      e. Administer I.V. heparin (treatment of choice if the source of the embolus is a clot) with initial bolus and maintenance by continuous drip or intermittent dosing for 7 to 10 days; administer oral anticoagulants concomitantly with heparin for 3 to 4 days before switching to oral agents alone
      f. Administer steroids to decrease local injury to tissue and to decrease pulmonary edema if the source is a fat embolus
      g. Monitor coagulation studies (partial thromboplastin time for heparin and prothrombin time for oral agents) to maintain levels at 1½ to 2 times normal values
      h. Obtain ABG measurements and monitor for hypoxemia and acid-base imbalances; monitor SaO_2 with pulse oximeter
      i. Position the patient for comfort; elevate the head of the bed to facilitate gas exchange; avoid bending at the knee
      j. Have the patient turn, cough, and deep-breathe to aid gas exchange and perfusion
      k. Avoid I.M. injections to decrease risk of hematoma
      l. Provide a safe environment to prevent falls and injury to tissue
      m. Monitor the patient for signs and symptoms of bleeding secondary to anticoagulant therapy
      n. Apply antiembolism stockings (remove at night and put on again before the patient ambulates in the morning) or use alternating-pressure devices with stockings continually if the patient is nonambulatory
      o. Prepare the patient for thrombolytic therapy with streptokinase or urokinase (used to speed lysis of clot, especially in hemodynamically compromised patients or those with large or multiple emboli)

p. Prepare the patient for embolectomy, which may be required to remove massive embolus; mortality rate of procedure exceeds 50%
q. Prepare the patient for surgical placement of a filter to prevent further movement of the thrombus (in selected patients)
r. Teach the patient the importance of preventing venous stasis by avoiding prolonged standing or sitting (especially with crossed legs) and avoiding the use of oral contraceptives
s. Teach the patient the importance of avoiding over-the-counter medications that may interfere with oral anticoagulant therapy

♦ VIII. Adult respiratory distress syndrome

A. General information
1. ARDS is noncardiogenic pulmonary edema caused by diffuse injury to the alveolar capillary membrane
2. It is known by other names, such as shock lung, white lung, and DaNang lung
3. ARDS mortality rate exceeds 50%
4. ARDS is characterized by phases, beginning with a precipitating event or insult that is followed by a progressive decrease in pulmonary compliance, decreased surfactant production, interstitial edema, refractory hypoxia, and widespread areas of consolidation

B. Causes
1. Trauma
2. Shock
3. Infection (especially gram-negative organisms)
4. Air embolism, fat embolism, or thromboembolism
5. Disseminated intravascular coagulopathy
6. Aspiration
7. Near drowning
8. Oxygen toxicity
9. Massive blood transfusions
10. Cardiopulmonary bypass

C. Assessment findings
1. Early
a. Labored breathing
b. Restlessness
c. Dry cough
d. Clear breath sounds
2. Late
a. Adventitious breath sounds
b. Cyanosis
c. Pallor

d. Agitation
e. Confusion
f. Accessory muscle retraction
g. Diaphoresis

D. Diagnostic test findings
1. Chest X-ray: normal in early phases; progressing to bilateral diffuse infiltrates, then to "whiteout," which is evidence of very little air in the lungs and characteristic of ARDS
2. Pulmonary function tests: decreased compliance and lung volume and elevated peak inspiratory pressures
3. ABG measurements: initially, respiratory alkalosis and hyperventilation; progresses to respiratory acidosis complicated by metabolic acidosis because of tissue hypoxia
4. Sputum analysis: elevated albumin level from leakage of serum albumin into the alveolar space
5. Hemodynamic monitoring: elevated pulmonary artery systolic and diastolic pressures but a normal PAWP

E. Patient care management
1. Goals
a. Maintain adequate arterial oxygenation and pulmonary ventilation
b. Treat the underlying disease
2. Strategies
a. Intubate and mechanically ventilate the patient to relieve the work of breathing (for more information about mechanical ventilation, see Chapter 7)
b. Administer oxygen therapy to correct hypoxia (may require a fraction of inspired oxygen [F_{IO_2}] of 50% or greater)

CLINICAL ALERT

(1) Monitor Sa_{O_2} with pulse oximeter
(2) Know that increasing hypoxia requiring higher F_{IO_2} and increased ventilatory pressures indicate that ARDS is progressing
c. Use positive end-expiratory pressure (PEEP) to maintain adequate P_{CO_2} (may require 20 cm H_2O or greater)
d. Suction as necessary to remove secretions
e. Administer a neuromuscular blocking agent, such as vecuronium bromide, to further decrease the work of breathing and maximize use of mechanical ventilation
f. Administer sedation with paralyzing drugs to decrease anxiety
g. Administer corticosteroids to assist in stabilizing the cell membrane, which decreases shift of proteins and fluid into the interstitium

h. Administer diuretic therapy to lower intravascular volume and to maintain a minimum PAWP to provide adequate CO
i. Administer fluid therapy of colloids for patients who are hypoalbuminemic and crystalloids for all others
j. Prepare the patient for pulmonary artery catheter placement to monitor fluid status and evaluate therapy
k. Assess and document CVP, PAP, PAWP, CO, and SVR
l. Assess and document continuous ECG rhythm; vital signs; mental status; heart, lung, and bowel sounds; urine output; and any signs and symptoms indicating changes in these parameters
m. Administer nutritional support to meet the patient's metabolic needs and defend against infection
n. Obtain ABG measurements and monitor for hypoxemia and acid-base imbalances; monitor SaO_2 with pulse oximeter
o. Position the patient for comfort; elevate the head of the bed to facilitate respiration
p. Have the patient turn, cough, and deep-breathe to aid gas exchange and perfusion
q. Schedule patient's activities between periods of rest to conserve energy and decrease oxygen demand
r. Provide emotional support to decrease fear and anxiety
s. Encourage the patient to cooperate with efforts to support breathing
t. Support the patient and family in their efforts to deal with the severity of the disease and the possibility of death

♦ IX. Exacerbation of chronic obstructive pulmonary disease (COPD)

A. General information
1. Exacerbation of COPD presents as an acute episode when the obstruction increases to the point of severe respiratory distress
2. If untreated, COPD leads to respiratory failure
3. Classification of COPD includes asthma (see "Status asthmaticus," pages 138 to 140); emphysema, which occurs because of decrease in lung elasticity, causing air trapping; and chronic bronchitis, which results from inflammation and excessive mucus production
4. COPD processes contribute to right ventricular failure and cor pulmonale
5. Patients with COPD are usually critically ill before they become symptomatic

B. Causes
1. Infection
2. Respiratory irritants or allergens
3. Cigarette smoking
4. Failure to take prescribed respiratory medications
5. Stress
6. Trauma

C. Assessment findings
1. Emphysema
   a. Nonproductive cough
   b Dyspnea
   c. Tachypnea
   d. Diminished lung sounds
   e. Use of accessory muscles for respiration
   f. Barrel chest
   g. Prolonged expiration
   h. Florid skin reflective of "pink puffer" syndrome
   i. Distant heart sounds
   j. Cachexia
2. Chronic bronchitis
   a. Productive cough with copious sputum
   b. Frequent infections
   c. Dyspnea
   d. Coarse wheezes and crackles
   e. Peripheral edema
   f. Ascites
   g. Increased neck vein distention
   h. Cyanosis reflective of "blue bloater" syndrome

D. Diagnostic test findings
1. Chest X-ray: hyperinflation with emphysema and congestion with bronchitis
2. Pulmonary function tests: increased functional residual volume and decreased vital capacity and expired volumes
3. ABG measurements: respiratory hypoxemia and respiratory acidosis
4. Sputum analysis for culture and sensitivity: identification of causative organism for appropriate antibiotic
5. ECG: right axis deviation and tachycardia

E. Patient care management
1. Goals
   a. Maintain adequate arterial oxygenation and pulmonary ventilation
   b. Treat underlying diseases

2. Strategies
   a. Administer oxygen therapy to treat hypoxia (may require a low flow rate of 1 to 2 liters/minute to prevent depression of hypoxic drive as stimulus to breathe)
   b. Intubate and mechanically ventilate the patient if he or she cannot maintain breathing (for more information on mechanical ventilation, see Chapter 7)
   c. Suction as necessary to remove secretions
   d. Use PEEP to lower FIO_2 and facilitate weaning from the ventilator; be aware that weaning may be more difficult because of increased retention of CO_2, which depresses the respiratory drive
   e. Prepare the patient for pulmonary artery catheter placement to monitor fluid status and evaluate therapy
   f. Assess and document CVP, PAP, PAWP, CO, PVR, and SVR
   g. Assess and document continuous ECG rhythm; vital signs; mental status; heart, lung, and bowel sounds; urine output; and any signs and symptoms indicating changes in these parameters
   h. Administer bronchodilators to dilate the smooth muscle of large airways
   i. Administer antibiotics appropriate for the causative organism if infection is present
   j. Administer corticosteroids to decrease inflammation
   k. Avoid the use of sedatives unless the patient is intubated and mechanically ventilated
   l. Administer I.V. fluids for hydration and medication therapy
   m. Provide nutritional support to meet the patient's metabolic needs and defend against infection
   n. Obtain ABG measurements and monitor for hypoxemia and acid-base imbalances; keep in mind that $PaCO_2$ may remain elevated and PaO_2 decreased, so baseline parameters should be established for comparison
   o. Monitor SaO_2 with pulse oximeter
   p. Position the patient for comfort; elevate the head of the bed to facilitate respiration
   q. Provide emotional support to decrease fear and anxiety
   r. Schedule patient's activities between periods of rest to conserve energy and decrease oxygen demands
   s. Teach the patient who smokes the importance of stopping smoking
   t. Teach the patient how to balance rest with activities
   u. Help the patient to recognize the signs and symptoms of exacerbation of the disease and the need for medical follow-up
   v. Teach the patient pursed-lip breathing to improve gas exchange

X. Tuberculosis (TB)

A. General information
1. TB is a necrotizing infection that most commonly involves the lungs
2. Reported cases have increased by 18% since 1981, largely due to immunosuppression such as human immunodeficiency virus (HIV)
3. Incidence is highest in those over age 65, except for people infected with HIV, which accelerates the disease
4. From 90% to 95% of those infected have latent disease that may become active after periods of stress
5. Outbreaks of multidrug-resistant TB (resistant to both isoniazid and rifampin) have become a serious concern because they have a high mortality
6. Triage should include vigorous efforts to detect patients with active disease

B. Causes
1. Inhalation of the microorganism *Mycobacterium tuberculosis* is the cause
2. Contributing factors include close exposure to infected people, other chronic diseases such as COPD, diabetes, infections, alcoholism, and other debilitating disease

C. Assessment findings
1. Common nonspecific symptoms
   a. Weight loss
   b. Fever (late evening)
   c. Night sweats
   d. Anorexia
   e. Malaise
2. Common pulmonary symptoms
   a. Cough with productive sputum
   b. Hemoptysis
   c. Pleuritic chest pain
   d. Adventitious breath sounds; crackles

D. Diagnostic test findings
1. Tuberculin skin test (purified protein derivative): positive if 10 mm or more of induration at 48 hours; 2 mm may be positive if patient is HIV-infected
2. Chest X-ray: peripheral infiltrates, cavitations
3. Sputum smear: highly suggestive of active disease if positive (immediate test results)
4. Sputum culture: diagnostic if positive (takes 4 weeks); sensitivity is done to identify appropriate drug therapy
5. WBC count and differential: usually normal

E. Patient care management
  1. Goal: to treat the infection and prevent its transmission to others
  2. Strategies
    a. Observe infection-control practices and isolation procedures, including airborne precautions (respiratory protection), until diagnosis is made and treatment with appropriate drug therapy results in negative sputum smears as defined by the Centers for Disease Control and Prevention and institutional policy
    b. Prevent transmission of infection by washing hands thoroughly and by wearing gloves when contact with blood or body fluids is likely
    c. Administer antibiotic regimen appropriate for the causative organism based on culture sensitivity
    d. Administer antipyretics for fever, as necessary
    e. Administer analgesics for pleuritic pain
    f. Monitor sputum production for color, viscosity, odor, and quantity
    g. Assess and document continuous ECG rhythm; vital signs; mental status; heart, lung, and bowel sounds; urine output; and signs and symptoms indicating changes in these parameters
    h. Hydrate with I.V. and oral fluids, but avoid overload
    i. Schedule activities between rest periods to conserve the patient's energy and decrease oxygen demand
    j. Teach the patient to prevent the spread of infection by covering his mouth and nose when coughing or sneezing and by properly disposing of soiled tissue and linens
    k. Help the patient identify the need for therapeutic assistance to stop smoking, if necessary

CLINICAL ALERT

    l. Know that TB is a reportable disease; all diagnosed cases and contacts must be reported to the local health department; patients must identify contacts likely to be exposed or infected so that treatment may be provided

POINTS TO REMEMBER

- Most patients in critical care or emergency areas have some degree of respiratory difficulty.
- Oxygen therapy should be used with caution in patients who depend on hypoxia for the stimulus to breathe.
- Narcotics depress the respiratory center.

- Critically ill patients may not be able to cough.
- Patients with chronic lung diseases may be critically ill before they become symptomatic.

STUDY QUESTIONS

To evaluate your understanding of this chapter, answer the following questions in the space provided; then compare your responses with the correct answers in Appendix B, pages 284 and 285.

1. What is the major management goal for a patient with a respiratory disorder? ______________________________

____

____

2. What is the normal stimulus for respiration? ______________________________

____

____

3. What characteristics of sputum should be observed for and documented?

____

____

4. Which auscultatory findings may be present in patients with status asthmaticus? ______________________________

____

____

5. What is the drug of choice for treating pulmonary embolus that is caused by a clot? ______________________________

____

____

6. Which auscultatory findings may be present in patients with emphysema?

____

____

7. Why are patients with COPD difficult to wean from mechanical ventilation? ______________________________

____

____

8. Which factors have contributed to the increase in TB in the past decade?

____

____

CRITICAL THINKING AND APPLICATION EXERCISES

1. Obtain 10 examples of ABGs from the laboratory, and analyze each for acid-base status and hypoxia.
2. Prepare a teaching plan for the patient and family to monitor forced expiratory volume in 1 second and peak expiratory flow rate for adequacy of asthma management.
3. Identify the type of SaO_2 monitor available in the clinical setting; describe to a classmate or an experienced nurse how the monitor determines saturation.
4. Compare and contrast "pink puffer" and "blue bloater" manifestations of COPD.
5. Observe a ventilation-perfusion ($\dot{V}/\dot{Q}$) scan, and describe to a classmate or an experienced nurse the significance of the findings.

CHAPTER

15

Metabolic and Renal Disorders

Learning objectives

After studying this chapter, you should be able to:

- Describe the general principles of metabolic and renal function.
- Identify possible causes for each type of alteration in metabolic or renal function.
- Discuss common assessment and diagnostic test findings for the patient with a specific alteration in metabolic or renal function.
- Describe care management for the patient with a specific alteration in metabolic or renal function.

Chapter overview

Caring for the patient with a metabolic or renal disorder in an emergency or critical care area requires a sound understanding of renal anatomy, physiology, and function. Various causes contribute to each type of alteration in metabolic or renal function. Common assessment and diagnostic test findings are used to determine the type and extent of dysfunction. Key regulatory functions of the renal system include acid excretion, electrolyte excretion, and water excretion. The kidneys also play an important role in blood pressure control, erythrocyte production, and vitamin D activation. The kidneys regulate metabolic processes and maintain a steady balance between acids and bases that ensures optimal functioning of the cells. For the kidneys to excrete metabolic waste adequately, three conditions must occur: the kidneys must be adequately perfused, they must function, and urine must be released from the body. In general, care management for a patient with a specific alteration in metabolic or renal function centers on treating the underlying cause of the dysfunction, correcting the metabolic disturbance, and minimizing the consequences of the dysfunction.

♦ I. Introduction

A. Functions
1. The kidneys' main function is to remove certain substances, including water, from the blood
2. The kidneys also play a key role in blood pressure control, calcium-phosphate metabolism, erythrocyte production, and vitamin D activation
3. The kidneys must be able to excrete substances that are digested and absorbed and not eliminated by other organs
4. Renal excretory function is necessary for the maintenance of life, but complete malfunction (unlike that of the cardiac and respiratory systems) may not cause death for several days. The renal system is adaptable to a wide variation in fluid load based on individual habits and patterns

B. Risk factors
1. Young or elderly people are particularly prone to fluid and electrolyte imbalances
2. Patients of any age with GI, renal, or skin losses are at risk for fluid and electrolyte losses
3. Patients who do not have access to water or who have an altered thirst mechanism, such as a comatose patient, are also prone to fluid and electrolyte imbalances
4. Patients with acute volume loss (such as from hemorrhage), those on certain antibiotics, those with coexisting medical conditions (such as congestive heart failure [CHF] or shock), and those with conditions that obstruct urine flow are at risk for developing renal failure

C. Potential nursing diagnoses for a patient with a metabolic or renal disorder
1. Fluid volume excess (related to fluid overload)
2. Fluid volume deficit (if caused by hypovolemia)
3. Altered nutrition: less than body requirements
4. Risk for infection

♦ II. Anatomy and physiology

A. Waste elimination

1. Key regulatory functions of the renal system include acid excretion, electrolyte excretion, and water excretion
2. For the kidneys to excrete metabolic waste adequately, three conditions must occur
   a. The kidneys must be adequately perfused
   b. They must function
   c. Urine must be released from the body
3. To excrete daily metabolic waste, normal kidneys must regulate renal blood flow at a constant level through autoregulatory mechanisms

CLINICAL ALERT

4. Normally, 20% to 25% of resting cardiac output (CO) is distributed to the kidneys; as the mean arterial pressure falls below 60 mm Hg, AUTOREGULATION may be overcome and the kidneys may become hypoperfused
5. Diminished blood flow damages kidney tissue, impairing function

B. Regulation of metabolic processes

1. The kidneys regulate metabolic processes and maintain a steady balance between acids and bases that ensures optimal functioning of the cells
   a. Acids are continuously liberated as metabolic by-products, yet the pH is kept within a narrow range
   b. The narrow pH is maintained by the body's buffer systems, which prevent large changes in pH by chemically combining acids with other ions
2. Metabolic acid-base imbalances are produced when the body cannot maintain a steady balance
3. Metabolic imbalances produce respiratory compensation, which begins in minutes

♦ III. Metabolic acidosis

A. General information

1. Metabolic acidosis is an acid-base imbalance that occurs when acids increase and the normal acid-base ratio of 1:20 is altered
2. Metabolic acidosis is not a disease but the result of increased acid production in the body or loss of bicarbonate (HCO_3^-)
3. Metabolic acidosis results from conditions that cause excessive fat metabolism in the absence of carbohydrates, anaerobic metabolism, underexcretion of metabolized acids, inability to conserve bases, and loss of HCO_3^- from the intestines

B. Causes
1. Diabetic ketoacidosis
2. Starvation
3. Renal failure
4. Poisoning
5. Diarrhea
6. Lactic acidosis
7. Intestinal fistulas
8. Administration of large amounts of normal saline solution or ammonium chloride

C. Assessment findings
1. Tachypnea (Kussmaul's respirations)
2. Headache
3. Confusion
4. Drowsiness
5. Cold, clammy skin

D. Diagnostic test findings
1. Arterial blood gas (ABG) measurements: uncompensated, pH less than 7.35, HCO_3^- less than 22 mEq/liter, Pa_{CO_2} normal; compensated, pH normal, HCO_3^- less than 22 mEq/liter, Pa_{CO_2} less than 35 mm Hg (for more information, see *Using ABGs to assess metabolic acid-base imbalances,* page 156)
2. Serum potassium: hyperkalemia
3. Urinalysis: decreased urine pH (depends on cause)
4. Electrocardiogram (ECG): arrhythmias from acidosis or hyperkalemia

E. Patient care management
1. Goal: to correct the metabolic defect
2. Strategies
   a. Administer drugs to treat the underlying pathophysiologic processes, such as insulin for diabetes
   b. Consider sodium bicarbonate administration to restore normal HCO_3^- levels
   c. Remember that hemodialysis may be indicated for severe metabolic disturbances that risk death
   d. Monitor ABG measurements and serum electrolyte levels as needed for changes, and document the patient's response to therapy
   e. Use continuous cardiac monitoring to detect cardiac rhythm disturbances
   f. Educate the patient and family about the risk factors and causative agents that should be modified, such as the misuse of medication or a delay in treating medical conditions

DECISION TREE

Using ABGs to assess metabolic acid-base imbalances

To help determine if a patient is experiencing a metabolic acid-base imbalance, follow the decision tree steps below to interpret the patient's ABGs.

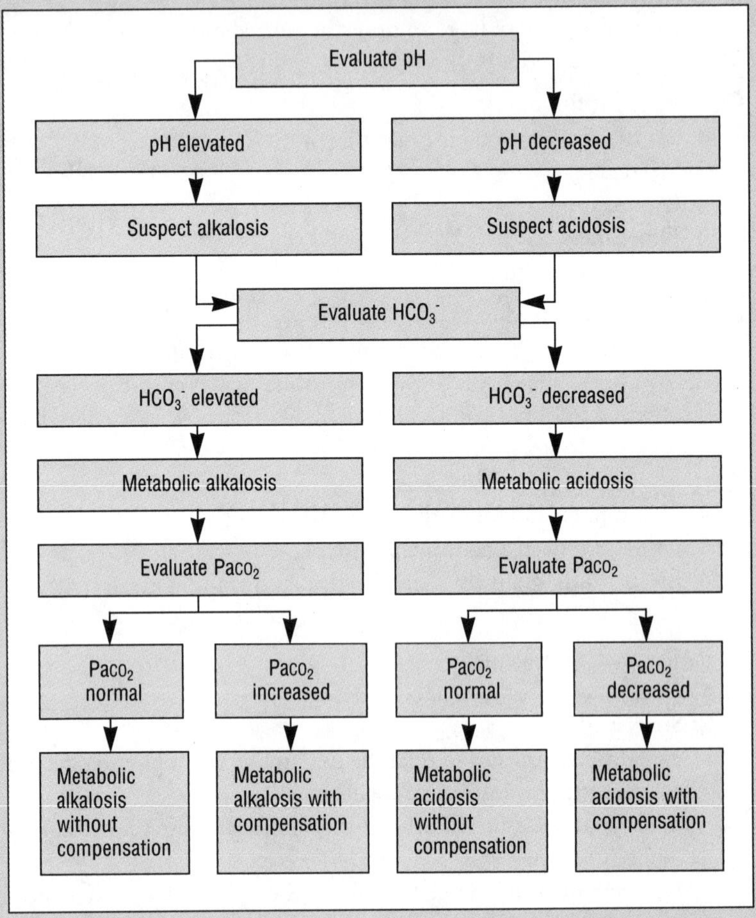

♦ IV. Metabolic alkalosis

A. General information

1. Metabolic alkalosis is an acid-base disturbance that occurs when bases increase and the normal acid-base ratio of 1:20 is altered
2. Metabolic alkalosis is not a disease but the result of decreased acids in the body or an increase in HCO_3^-

3. Metabolic alkalosis is produced from conditions that cause severe acid loss, decreased serum potassium and chloride, and excessive HCO_3^- intake

B. Causes
1. Vomiting
2. GI suctioning
3. Diuretic therapy
4. Cushing's syndrome
5. Excessive antacid ingestion

C. Assessment findings
1. Increased neuromuscular irritability
2. Numbness or tingling of fingers and toes
3. Tetany
4. Seizures
5. Arrhythmias
6. Hypoventilation

D. Diagnostic test findings
1. ABG measurements: uncompensated, pH greater than 7.45, HCO_3^- greater than 26 mEq/liter, $Paco_2$ normal; compensated, pH normal, HCO_3^- greater than 26 mEq/liter, $Paco_2$ greater than 45 mm Hg
2. Serum electrolytes: decreased potassium, calcium, and chloride
3. Urine electrolytes: decreased chloride
4. ECG: arrhythmias from alkalosis or hypokalemia

E. Patient care management
1. Goal: to correct the metabolic defect
2. Strategies
   a. Administer drugs to treat underlying pathophysiologic processes, such as antiemetics for vomiting
   b. Infuse I.V. normal saline solution to replace fluid volume and chloride
   c. Administer potassium chloride to correct electrolyte imbalances
   d. Monitor ABG measurements and serum and urine electrolytes frequently for changes, and document the patient's response to therapy
   e. Use continuous cardiac monitoring to detect cardiac rhythm disturbances
   f. Educate the patient and family about the risk factors and causative agents that should be modified, such as the misuse of medication or a delay in the treatment of medical conditions

♦ V. Electrolyte disturbances

A. General information
1. Electrolyte disturbances occur when extracellular electrolyte concentrations fall outside normal levels
2. Electrolytes serve many functions within the body, such as assisting with regulation of water and acid-base balance, affecting neuromuscular activity, and contributing to enzyme reactions
3. As the electrolyte balance is disturbed, alterations in body functions occur
4. The major electrolytes are sodium, potassium, calcium, and magnesium
5. Concentrations of intracellular and extracellular electrolytes differ: sodium is more abundant in extracellular fluid (ECF), whereas potassium is concentrated in intracellular fluid (ICF)

CLINICAL ALERT

6. Serum levels of electrolytes measure extracellular concentrations but may not always provide an accurate index of intracellular levels
7. ECG changes are the most reliable indicators of potassium levels

B. Causes: see *Electrolyte disturbances* for specific information

C. Assessment findings
1. An electrolyte imbalance reflects body function disturbances
2. Signs and symptoms become more severe as electrolyte imbalances worsen (see *Electrolyte disturbances* for specific information)

D. Diagnostic test findings
1. Serum levels of electrolytes: increased or decreased
2. ABG measurements: acid-base disturbances
3. ECG with hypokalemia: flattened T wave, depressed ST segment, prominent U wave
4. ECG with hyperkalemia: widened QRS complex; tall, tented T wave; flattened P wave; depressed ST segment; prolonged PR interval; and asystole
5. ECG with hypercalcemia: arrhythmias and shortened QT interval
6. ECG with hypocalcemia: prolonged QT interval
7. ECG with hypermagnesemia: widened QRS complex, prolonged PR interval, elevated T wave
8. ECG with hypomagnesemia: flattened T wave, slight widening of QRS complex, diminished voltage of P waves and QRS complex, prominent U wave

E. Patient care management
1. Goals
   a. Correct the underlying cause of the electrolyte imbalance
   b. Return the electrolyte level to normal (see *Electrolyte disturbances*, pages 159 and 160, for specific management)

Electrolyte disturbances

ELECTROLYTE DISTURBANCE	CAUSES	ASSESSMENT FINDINGS	PATIENT CARE MANAGEMENT
Hyponatremia (sodium [Na] < 135 mEq/liter)	GI, skin, or renal losses; syndrome of inappropriate antidiuretic hormone; congestive heart failure; oliguric renal failure; liver failure; inadequate sodium intake; excess water intake or retention; burns; hemorrhage	Abdominal and muscle cramps, anorexia, headache, postural hypotension, lethargy, confusion, seizures	Administer I.V. hypertonic saline solution (3% or 5% sodium chloride); initiate seizure precautions and other safety measures
Hypernatremia (Na > 145 mEq/liter)	Osmotic diuresis, diabetes insipidus, saltwater near drowning, inability to perceive thirst, high-protein feedings; inadequate water intake	Low-grade fever; flushed skin; weakness; thirst; hypotension; pulmonary congestion; edema; dry, swollen tongue; disorientation	Administer water I.V. or by mouth to replace loss. Give diuretics and water I.V. or by mouth for sodium gain; correct slowly to prevent cerebral edema
Hypokalemia (potassium [K] < 3 mEq/liter)	GI or renal losses, hyperaldosteronism, increased diaphoresis, diuretics, diabetic ketoacidosis	Fatigue, nausea, vomiting, muscle weakness, decreased bowel motility, anorexia; hyporeflexia; cardiac arrhythmias	Administer K I.V. or by mouth for replacement; administer parenterally, not to exceed 40 mEq/2-hr period; institute cardiac monitoring
Hyperkalemia (K > 5.5 mEq/liter)	Renal disease, potassium-sparing diuretics, tissue breakdown, acidosis, insulin deficiency, excessive potassium replacement, lead poisoning, burns	Muscle weakness, nausea, diarrhea, hypotension, cardiac arrhythmias	Give ion exchange resin to exchange Na for K. Give I.V. glucose insulin and sodium bicarbonate ($NaHCO_3$) to drive K into cell temporarily. Give I.V. calcium (Ca) gluconate to block neuromuscular and cardiac effects. Institute cardiac monitoring

(continued)

Electrolyte disturbances *(continued)*

ELECTROLYTE DISTURBANCE	CAUSES	ASSESSMENT FINDINGS	PATIENT CARE MANAGEMENT
Hypocalcemia (calcium [Ca] < 8.5 mg/dl)	Alkalosis, administration of banked citrated blood, impaired vitamin D absorption, hypoparathyroidism, decreased magnesium or phosphate; overuse of laxatives containing phosphates	Tetany, seizures, positive Chvostek's and Trousseau's signs, tingling of fingers and mouth, muscular twitching, memory impairment, seizures, cardiac arrhythmias	Give Ca I.V. or by mouth for replacement. Give vitamin D by mouth to increase GI absorption of Ca. Give aluminum hydroxide by mouth to promote binding with phosphate. Institute seizure precautions and cardiac monitoring
Hypercalcemia (Ca > 10.5 mg/dl)	Acidosis, renal failure, cancer or multiple myeloma, hyperparathyroidism, increased intestinal absorption, excessive calcium intake orally or in solution, immobility, osteoporosis	Muscle weakness, nausea, vomiting, anorexia, constipation, memory impairment, abdominal pain, cardiac arrhythmias	Administer normal saline solution I.V. to aid Ca excretion. Give phosphate I.V. to cause inverse drop in Ca. Encourage low-calcium diet. Administer steroids to alter vitamin D absorption. Promote weight bearing, if tolerated, to stimulate bone deposition. Give $NaHCO_3$ to treat acidosis. Begin cardiac monitoring
Hypomagnesemia (magnesium [Mg] < 1.5 mEq/liter)	Alcoholism, GI loss, administration of banked citrated blood, osmotic diuresis, hypercalcemia, elevated aldosterone levels, hyperthyroidism, acute pancreatitis, diabetic ketoacidosis	Tremors, difficulty swallowing, tetany, positive Chvostek's and Trousseau's signs, seizures, mood swings, hyperreflexia, cardiac arrhythmias	Increase dietary intake of Ca. Administer magnesium sulfate I.V., and observe for signs of hypermagnesemia. Institute cardiac monitoring and seizure precautions
Hypermagnesemia (Mg > 2.5 mEq/liter)	Renal failure, excessive Mg administration, untreated diabetic ketoacidosis, severe dehydration, excessive infusion of magnesium-containing fluids	Facial flushing, hypotension, respiratory depression, muscle weakness, loss of deep tendon reflexes, cardiac arrhythmias, coma	Administer Ca I.V. Prepare for dialysis. Institute mechanical ventilation if respiratory depression is significant. Institute cardiac monitoring

2. Strategies
   a. Monitor intake and output to assess fluid status
   b. Monitor ECG to observe for signs of continuing changes in cardiac rhythm or complexes
   c. Carefully reposition the patient with hypercalcemia because bones may be brittle and fractures are possible
   d. Assess the patient with hypercalcemia for signs and symptoms of kidney stone formation, such as hematuria, intermittent low back pain, and nausea or vomiting
   e. Ensure that the patient with hypomagnesemia can swallow before administering oral medications or foods
   f. Evaluate the patient with hypermagnesemia for decreased deep tendon reflexes

CLINICAL ALERT

   g. Be alert for the need of emergency intervention or mechanical ventilation if the patient develops respiratory depression from hypermagnesemia
   h. Teach the patient to avoid over-the-counter medications that contribute to electrolyte imbalance
   i. Document the patient's response to therapy

♦ VI. Fluid volume disturbances

A. General information
   1. Fluid volume disturbances are alterations in the normal fluid balance within the body
   2. Fluid disturbances can be caused by disease, illness-related changes in ingestion of fluid or food, or therapy
   3. In the critically ill patient, the kidneys and other organs responsible for regulating fluid and electrolytes often fail, complicating the disturbance
   4. When the compensatory mechanisms fail, the nurse plays a crucial role in calculating fluid gain or loss and administering fluid volume precisely

CLINICAL ALERT

   5. Failure to properly recognize and treat fluid disturbances in the critically ill patient can produce fatal complications
   6. Fluid volume disturbances are of two major types: fluid volume excess and fluid volume deficit
      a. *Fluid volume excess* reflects an increased accumulation of water and electrolytes in the ECF; it usually results from an increase in total sodium concentration, causing more water to be drawn into the ECF to reestablish the proper sodium-water ratio
      b. *Fluid volume deficit* results from excessive loss of water and electrolytes from ECF

7. Fluid volume deficit may be *isotonic* (sodium and water are lost in equal proportions), *hypertonic* (more water than sodium is lost or ECF concentration of sodium increases), or *hypotonic* (more sodium than water is lost or ECF concentration of water increases)

B. Causes
1. Fluid volume excess
   a. Fluid overload
   b. Sodium overload
   c. Diminished homeostatic mechanisms, such as those occurring in CHF, cirrhosis, or excessive corticosteroid therapy
2. Fluid volume deficit
   a. Insufficient intake of water and electrolytes
   b. Excessive fluid loss through secretions or excretions
   c. Both conditions occurring simultaneously (most common)
   d. Third-space shifting

C. Assessment findings
1. Fluid volume excess
   a. Excessive weight gain (1 liter of fluid weighs about 2¼ lb [1 kg])
   b. Elevated blood pressure
   c. Dyspnea
   d. Neck vein distention
   e. Elevated central venous pressure (CVP)
   f. Elevated pulmonary artery pressure (PAP)
   g. Dependent edema; may be pitting
   h. Bounding pulses
   i. Crackles
2. Fluid volume deficit
   a. Oliguria
   b. Dizziness
   c. Syncope
   d. Poor skin turgor
   e. Dry mucous membranes
   f. Hypotension
   g. Orthostatic blood pressure differences
   h. Decreased CVP, PAP, and CO
   i. Weakness
   j. Nausea and vomiting

D. Diagnostic test findings
1. Fluid volume excess (related to hemodilution)
   a. Blood urea nitrogen (BUN) level: decreased
   b. Complete blood count (CBC): decreased hematocrit (HCT) levels

c. Serum sodium: normal or decreased
d. Serum and urine osmolality: decreased in patients with normal renal function

2. Fluid volume deficit (related to hemoconcentration; may vary with type of fluid volume deficit)
   a. BUN-creatinine ratio: greater than normal ratio of 10:1
   b. CBC: increased HCT levels
   c. Serum sodium: increased (hypertonic), decreased (hypotonic), or normal (isotonic)
   d. Serum and urine osmolality: increased (hypertonic), decreased (hypotonic), or normal (isotonic)
   e. Urine specific gravity: elevated (may not occur for several hours)

E. Patient care management
1. Goals
   a. Restore normal fluid volume to ECF
   b. Treat causative factors
2. Strategies for fluid volume excess
   a. Administer diuretics to decrease fluid volume
   b. Maintain fluid restrictions to promote fluid balance
   c. Discontinue sodium-containing fluids to prevent further fluid retention
   d. Provide sodium-restricted diet to prevent further fluid retention
   e. Consider dialysis or continuous renal replacement therapies (CRRT) to quickly correct fluid overload
   f. Monitor intake and output hourly for changes
   g. Assess hemodynamic parameters, especially CVP and PAP, for changes
   h. Measure urine specific gravity as needed to evaluate the patient's fluid status and response to therapy

CLINICAL ALERT

   i. Weigh the patient daily at the same time and on the same scale with patient wearing the same amount of clothing to evaluate fluid balance
   j. Monitor for signs of pulmonary edema, such as shortness of breath and dyspnea
   k. Evaluate for possible causative factors, such as heart failure, renal failure, burns, excessive glucocorticoid administration, and overzealous administration of I.V. fluids
3. Strategies for fluid volume deficit
   a. Administer dextrose 5% in water (D_5W) for replacement; D_5W provides 170 calories/liter and shifts evenly between ICF and ECF
   b. Consider administering normal saline solution (0.9% sodium chloride) to expand ECF only because it is an isotonic fluid that corrects mild sodium depletion

c. Use albumin to expand the intravascular component of ECF and pull fluid into blood vessels from interstitial spaces
d. Give blood to expand the intravascular component of ECF
e. Consider vasopressors when the patient is adequately hydrated but response to volume replacement is inadequate
f. Monitor intake and output hourly to assess fluid balance accurately
g. Assess hemodynamic parameters, especially CVP, PAP, and CO
h. Measure urine specific gravity as needed to evaluate the patient's fluid status and response to therapy

CLINICAL ALERT

i. Weigh the patient daily at the same time and on the same scale with the same amount of linens or clothes to ensure accurate measurements
j. Institute safety measures to prevent injury to the patient with altered sensorium
k. Evaluate for possible causative factors, such as GI, skin, or renal losses; third-space shifting; altered intake; and hemorrhage

♦ VII. Acute renal failure (ARF)

A. General information

1. ARF is a sudden deterioration in kidney function that results from the kidneys' inability to excrete water and metabolic wastes, leading to a progressive rise in creatinine and urea levels
2. Renal failure is classified as prerenal, intrarenal, or postrenal, based on the underlying cause of failure
   a. *Prerenal* renal failure is caused by low perfusion to the kidneys
   b. *Intrarenal* renal failure is caused by damage to the kidneys
   c. *Postrenal* renal failure is caused by an obstruction between the kidneys and the urinary meatus
3. ARF can have a dramatic effect on fluid and electrolyte and acid-base balances
4. The most common cause of ARF is acute tubular necrosis
5. The key to ARF prevention is assessment of the patient at risk, including elderly, obese, or female patients and those with underlying renal problems, chronic illness, or recent infections

CLINICAL ALERT

6. Certain drugs, primarily those excreted by the kidneys, require dosage modification in patients with ARF

B. Causes

1. Prerenal
   a. Impaired cardiac function
   b. Hypovolemia
   c. Peripheral vasodilation

   d. Renal vascular obstruction
   e. Use of vasconstrictors
2. Intrarenal
   a. NEPHROTOXIC drugs
   b. Infection
   c. Pigment release, such as sepsis, transfusion reactions
   d. Rhabdomyolysis
   e. Obstetric complications, such as eclampsia, septic abortion
   f. Other parenchymal disorders
   g. Prerenal conditions
3. Postrenal
   a. Ureteral obstruction
   b. Bladder obstruction
   c. Urethral obstruction (prostatic hypertrophy)

C. Assessment findings

1. Decreased urine output (less than 400 ml/day) for 1 to 2 weeks, followed by diuresis sometimes exceeding 3 liters/day for 2 to 4 weeks, with a recovery period of up to 1 year
2. Weakness
3. Increased blood pressure
4. Arrhythmias
5. Kussmaul's respirations
6. Peripheral edema
7. Bleeding tendencies
8. GI disturbances, such as anorexia, nausea, and vomiting
9. Changes in level of consciousness, such as behavioral changes and confusion
10. Muscle irritability
11. Weight gain
12. Pallor

D. Diagnostic test findings

1. Serum chemistry: increased BUN, creatinine, potassium, phosphorus, and magnesium levels; decreased calcium, carbon dioxide, and sodium levels
2. BUN-creatinine ratio: prerenal, greater than 20:1; intrarenal, 10:1; postrenal, 10:1
3. Urine sodium: decreased (prerenal), increased (intrarenal), or normal (postrenal)
4. Urine osmolality: increased (prerenal), decreased (intrarenal), or normal (postrenal)

5. Urine specific gravity: increased (prerenal), fixed at 1.010 (intrarenal), or normal (postrenal)
6. Urine sediment: normal (prerenal), casts and proteinuria (intrarenal), crystals (postrenal)
7. CBC: decreased HCT and hemoglobin levels and red blood cell count; increased prothrombin time and partial thromboplastin time
8. ABG measurements: decreased pH and HCO_3^-
9. Creatinine clearance test: less than 50 ml/minute
10. Kidneys, ureter, and bladder and flat plate of abdomen X-rays: rules out renal obstruction as a cause
11. Excretory urography: rules out complete or partial urinary system obstruction
12. Renal scan: decreased perfusion to the kidneys
13. Renal failure index: prerenal less than 1; intrarenal greater than 1
14. Fraction of excreted sodium: prerenal less than 1; intrarenal greater than 1

E. Patient care management
1. Goals
   a. Treat underlying cause
   b. Correct metabolic disturbances
2. Strategies
   a. Assess and document continuous ECG rhythm; vital signs; mental status; heart, lung, and bowel sounds; urine output; and any signs or symptoms indicating changes in these parameters
   b. Weigh the patient daily at the same time and on the same scale with the same amount of linens or clothes
   c. Administer I.V. fluid therapy to correct fluid volume and electrolyte imbalances
   d. Administer low-dose dopamine (prerenal) to increase blood pressure and CO volume
   e. Assess for signs of fluid overload or hypovolemic shock
   f. Monitor serum chemistry for electrolyte imbalances
   g. Anticipate the need for I.V. calcium gluconate to counteract the toxic cardiac effects of hyperkalemia
   h. Administer cation exchange resins, such as sodium polystyrene sulfonate, orally or rectally to lower serum potassium levels by removing potassium through the GI tract
   i. Administer diuretic therapy after the patient is adequately hydrated (prerenal)
   j. Determine the causative agent of intrarenal ARF, and discontinue any related antibiotics, analgesics, anesthetics, or pesticide exposure

TEACHING TIPS

Patient recovering from ARF

Be sure to include the following topics in your teaching plan for a patient recovering from acute renal failure (ARF).

- Signs and symptoms necessitating medical attention, including signs and symptoms of urinary tract infection and decreased urine output
- Importance of complying with treatment, including dietary restrictions
- Activation of emergency medical system, if needed
- Medication regimen, including dosage, scheduling, and adverse effects
- Avoidance of over-the-counter (OTC) drugs without first checking with the doctor (many OTC drugs are high in sodium)
- Monitoring for patency of the vascular access device, if present
- Lifestyle changes to minimize behaviors or activities that aggravate the patient's condition

k. Institute dietary restrictions — including a diet low in protein, potassium, and sodium and high in carbohydrates — either orally, enterally, or parenterally

l. Administer blood products to stabilize HCT and platelet count (intrarenal)

m. Administer antibiotic therapy to treat the urinary tract infection, if present (postrenal)

n. Prepare for possible dialysis or CRRT if interventions are unsuccessful

o. Educate the patient about the disorder and its treatment (for specific teaching tips, see *Patient recovering from ARF*)

p. Document the patient's response to therapy

POINTS TO REMEMBER

- The renal system is responsible for regulating excretion of water, electrolytes, and acid substances.
- A mean arterial pressure of 60 mm Hg is necessary for renal system autoregulation.
- Metabolic acid-base imbalances are caused by an underlying disease that disrupts the normal acid-base ratio.
- Major electrolyte imbalances can be life-threatening.

- The most reliable indicators of ECF potassium imbalances are ECG changes.
- The most common cause of ARF is acute tubular necrosis.
- Prevention of ARF is a primary goal in susceptible patients.

STUDY QUESTIONS

To evaluate your understanding of this chapter, answer the following questions in the space provided; then compare your responses with the correct answers in Appendix B, page 285.

1. What are the three key functions of the renal system? ____________

2. What are two common causes of metabolic acidosis? ____________

3. Which ABG findings differentiate uncompensated metabolic acidosis from compensated metabolic acidosis? ____________

4. What is the most reliable indicator of potassium imbalance? ____________

5. Which ECG changes are found in electrolyte imbalances? ____________

6. What are the common causes of fluid volume deficit? ____________

7. What is the most common cause of ARF? ____________

Critical Thinking and Application Exercises

1. Develop a chart comparing the major drugs used for treating hyperkalemia.
2. Follow a patient with ARF from admission through discharge. Develop a plan of care, including any need for follow-up and home care.
3. Develop a presentation for your classmates describing the major drugs causing nephrotoxicity. Describe how to obtain a peak and trough blood specimen and the rationale behind these tests.
4. List two strategies that can be used to enhance safety in a patient with hypernatremia.
5. Develop a chart that shows the differences among prerenal, intrarenal, and postrenal failure in relation to cause, pathophysiology, and patient care management.

CHAPTER

16

Endocrine Disorders

Learning objectives

After studying this chapter, you should be able to:

- Describe the general principles of endocrine function.
- Identify possible causes for each type of alteration in endocrine function.
- Discuss common assessment and diagnostic test findings for the patient with a specific endocrine disorder.
- Describe care management for the patient with a specific alteration in endocrine function.

Chapter overview

Caring for the patient with an endocrine disorder requires an understanding of endocrine anatomy and physiology. A thorough assessment is essential to planning and implementing care. The assessment includes a history, identification of causes and risk factors, examination for signs and symptoms, and diagnostic test findings. Nursing diagnoses focus primarily on alteration in tissue perfusion, fluid volume deficit or excess, alteration in nutrition, and sensory or perceptual alterations. The major goals of patient care management are to restore normal hormone production, secretion, or utilization and to minimize the detrimental effects of hormonal imbalance on the body.

♦ I. Introduction

A. Function
   1. The endocrine system regulates secretion of HORMONES that alter metabolic body functions
      a. Chemical reactions
      b. Growth
      c. Transport of chemicals
   2. Treatment involves restoring normal hormone production or secretion

B. Risk factors
   1. Injury to any organ of the system
   2. Injury to the nervous system, which controls the endocrine system by means of feedback mechanisms
   3. Genetic or hereditary mechanisms
   4. Age: elderly patients have an increased risk

C. Potential nursing diagnoses for a patient with endocrine system dysfunction
   1. Altered tissue perfusion
   2. Fluid volume deficit or excess
   3. Altered nutrition
   4. Sensory or perceptual alterations

♦ II. Anatomy and physiology

A. Regulation
   1. The endocrine system is closely related to the nervous system for regulation and control of specific hormones through its feedback systems
   2. Feedback systems involve the hypothalamus, pituitary gland, and target glands

B. Hormones
   1. Hormones, released directly into the bloodstream, act as chemical messengers
   2. They act directly on the target organ
   3. They have a generalized effect on the entire body

C. Dysfunction
   1. Endocrine dysfunction involves either insufficient or excessive hormone production or secretion from a variety of causes
   2. Possible causes
      a. Congenital or genetic defects
      b. Surgery
      c. Atrophy
      d. Neoplasms

♦ III. Diabetic ketoacidosis (DKA)

A. General information
   1. DKA is an emergency condition of hyperglycemia and KETONEMIA resulting from deficient insulin production or the cells' inability to use insulin
   2. DKA is the most common complication of DIABETES MELLITUS
   3. In the absence of glucose, fat is broken down for energy; this results in ketonuria and ketonemia
   4. DKA can lead to severe dehydration and electrolyte depletion from osmotic diuresis, metabolic acidosis from hyperketonemia, and hyperosmolarity from hyperglycemia and dehydration
   5. Signs and symptoms develop quickly and require prompt attention
   6. Phagocytosis is impaired with serum glucose levels equal to or greater than 200 mg/dl, which can delay wound healing and predispose the patient to infection

B. Causes
   1. History of uncontrolled insulin-dependent diabetes mellitus (Type I)

CLINICAL ALERT

   2. Infection
      a. Although the stress of an infection increases the need for glucose utilization, many diabetic patients do not take their daily insulin doses when they have cold and flu symptoms because their appetite is decreased
      b. This results in hyperglycemia, despite the decrease in oral intake
   3. Surgery
   4. Trauma
   5. Stress
   6. Pregnancy
   7. Decreased exercise
   8. Increased food intake without appropriate insulin adjustment
   9. Inadequate exogenous insulin administration

C. Assessment findings
   1. Dry, flushed skin
   2. Dehydration, evidenced by dry mucous membranes and poor skin turgor
   3. Fruity breath odor
   4. Kussmaul's respirations (rapid and deep)
   5. POLYPHAGIA, polydipsia, or polyuria
   6. Fever
   7. Nausea, vomiting, or abdominal pain
   8. Altered level of consciousness (LOC) from irritability progressing to coma

D. Diagnostic test findings

1. Serum glucose level: 200 to 800 mg/dl
2. Serum ketone level: elevated
3. Urine ketone level: elevated
4. Serum sodium level: decreased
5. Serum potassium level: elevated initially, then decreased because of diuresis and reversal of acidosis
6. Arterial blood gas (ABG) measurements: pH reflects acidosis
7. Hemoglobin (Hb) and hematocrit (HCT) levels: elevated because of diuresis and dehydration
8. Hemodynamic monitoring: pressures below the patient's normal baseline reflect dehydration
9. Electrocardiogram (ECG): arrhythmias from potassium imbalance

E. Patient care management

1. Goals
   a. Hydrate patient
   b. Restore acid-base balance
2. Strategies
   a. Administer regular insulin first as a bolus, then as a continuous I.V. infusion to decrease serum glucose level
   b. Administer I.V. fluids to correct dehydration (usually 0.9% or 0.45% saline solution); initially given rapidly until serum glucose levels decrease to 200 to 300 mg/dl; then administer glucose solutions to prevent hypoglycemia caused by insulin administration
   c. Administer fluids through a large-bore peripheral I.V. line to allow for rapid infusion
   d. Monitor serum electrolytes: sodium, potassium, phosphate, and calcium
   e. Administer I.V. potassium to replace serum potassium that returns to the intracellular fluid with the reversal of acidosis
   f. Prepare the patient for pulmonary artery catheter placement to monitor fluid status and evaluate therapy
   g. Assess and document central venous pressure (CVP), pulmonary artery pressure (PAP), pulmonary artery wedge pressure (PAWP), cardiac output (CO), and systemic vascular resistance (SVR)
   h. Assess and document continuous ECG rhythm; vital signs; mental status; heart, lung, and bowel sounds; urine output; and any signs and symptoms indicating changes in these parameters
   i. Insert a nasogastric (NG) tube to relieve gastric distention and prevent aspiration if gag reflex is absent
   j. Administer antibiotics to treat the underlying infection, if present

k. Monitor and report abnormalities in serum glucose and electrolyte levels
l. Obtain ABG measurements and monitor for hypoxemia and acid-base imbalance; monitor arterial oxygen saturation (SaO_2) with a pulse oximeter
m. Provide safety measures to prevent accidental injury from altered LOC
n. Position the patient for comfort; elevate the head of the bed to facilitate respiration and prevent aspiration
o. Teach the patient the causes of DKA
p. Teach the patient to recognize signs and symptoms of hyperglycemia requiring medical intervention
q. Instruct the patient in the proper technique for insulin administration and blood glucose testing to monitor diabetes, and have the patient demonstrate the technique

♦ IV. Hyperosmolar hyperglycemic nonketotic syndrome (HHNS)

A. General information
1. HHNS is a life-threatening emergency caused by severe hyperglycemia but with an absence of ketone production
2. Insulin is present in amounts adequate to prevent ketosis but not hyperglycemia
3. Hyperglycemia is usually more pronounced in HHNS than in DKA (for more information, see *Distinguishing between DKA and HHNS*)
4. The mortality rate from HHNS ranges from 25% to 50%
5. HHNS primarily occurs in elderly patients with no history of diabetes

CLINICAL ALERT

6. Signs and symptoms may develop gradually, taking up to 2 weeks to become severe, and typically are nonspecific
7. Elderly patients commonly do not manifest acute clinical symptoms of illness and can become critically ill before symptoms are recognized; this increases their risk of morbidity and mortality

B. Causes
1. Undiagnosed non-insulin-dependent diabetes mellitus (Type II)
2. Stress
3. Infection
4. Acute pancreatitis
5. Alcohol ingestion
6. Trauma, such as head injury and burns
7. Failure of thirst mechanism with subsequent lack of oral intake

DECISION TREE

Distinguishing between DKA and HHNS

Diabetic ketoacidosis (DKA) and hyperosmolar hyperglycemic nonketotic syndrome (HHNS) are two acute complications of diabetes. Use the decision tree below to help distinguish between these two complications when assessing the patient.

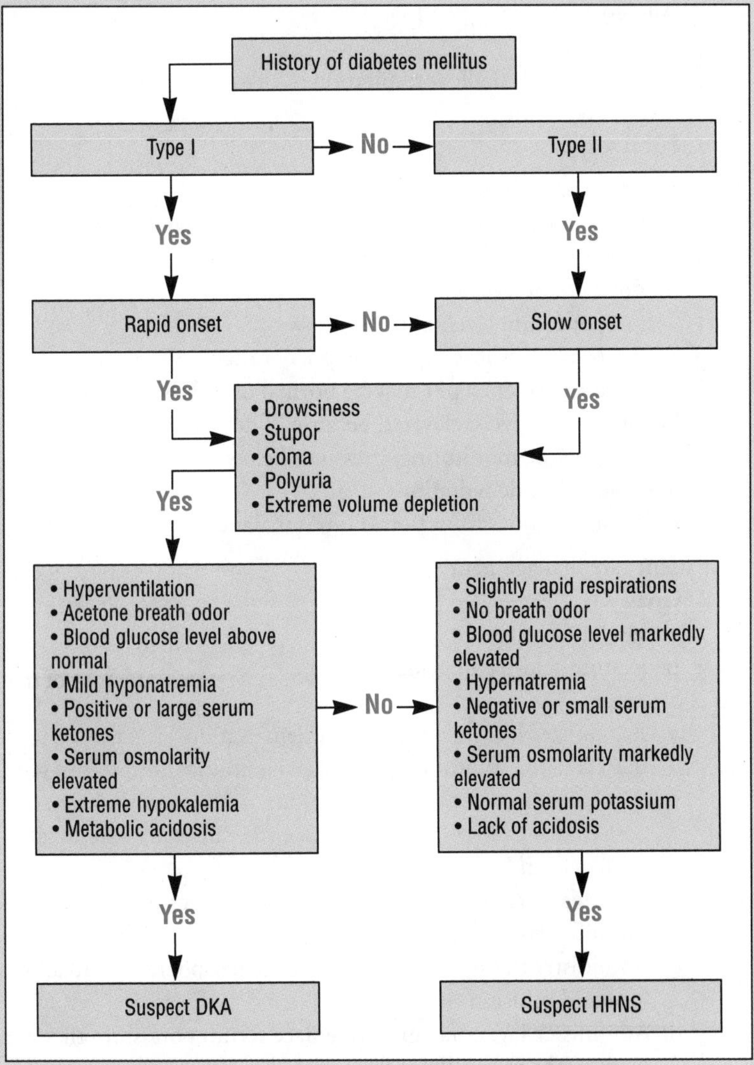

8. Medical therapy, such as total parenteral nutrition, peritoneal dialysis, and hypothermia
9. Medications, such as glucocorticoids, phenytoin, and diuretics

C. Assessment findings
1. Severe dehydration, evidenced by dry mucous membranes and poor skin turgor
2. Polydipsia and polyuria
3. Altered LOC
4. Hypotension
5. Tachypnea with shallow respirations
6. Profound weakness
7. Focal seizures

D. Diagnostic test findings
1. Serum glucose level: elevated (may be greater than 800 mg/dl)
2. Urinalysis: absence of ketonuria
3. Serum sodium level: elevated
4. Serum potassium level: normal or low
5. Serum osmolality level: elevated (greater than 350 mOsm/liter)
6. ABG measurements: pH may be normal or mildly acidotic
7. Hb and HCT levels: elevated because of dehydration
8. Hemodynamic monitoring: pressures below the patient's normal baseline reflect dehydration
9. ECG: arrhythmias from potassium imbalance

E. Patient care management
1. Goals
   a. Hydrate patient
   b. Restore acid-base balance
2. Strategies
   a. Administer I.V. fluids to correct dehydration (usually 0.9% or 0.45% saline solution); initially given rapidly until serum glucose levels decrease to 200 to 300 mg/dl; then administer glucose solutions to prevent hypoglycemia caused by insulin administration
   b. Administer regular insulin first as a bolus, then as a continuous I.V. infusion to decrease serum glucose concentration
   c. Administer fluids through a large-bore peripheral I.V. to allow for rapid infusion
   d. Administer I.V. potassium to replace serum potassium that returns to the intracellular fluid with the reversal of hyperosmolality
   e. Prepare the patient for pulmonary artery catheter placement to monitor fluid status and evaluate therapy
   f. Assess and document CVP, PAP, PAWP, CO, and SVR

g. Assess and document continuous ECG rhythm; vital signs; mental status; heart, lung, and bowel sounds; urine output; and any signs and symptoms indicating changes in these parameters
h. Insert an NG tube to relieve gastric distention and prevent aspiration if gag reflex is absent
i. Administer antibiotics to treat the underlying infection, if present
j. Monitor and report abnormalities in serum glucose and electrolyte levels
k. Obtain ABG measurements and monitor for hypoxemia and acid-base imbalance; monitor SaO_2 with pulse oximeter
l. Provide safety measures to prevent accidental injury from altered LOC
m. Position the patient for comfort; elevate the head of the bed to facilitate respiration and prevent aspiration
n. Teach the patient to recognize signs and symptoms of hyperglycemia requiring medical intervention
o. Instruct the patient in the proper technique for blood glucose testing to monitor diabetes, and have the patient demonstrate the technique

♦ V. Hypoglycemia

A. General information
1. Hypoglycemia is an emergency situation in which serum glucose levels fall below 50 mg/dl
2. Normal homeostatic mechanisms maintain serum glucose levels at 60 to 100 mg/dl
3. Signs and symptoms appear suddenly and require immediate action to correct
4. Hypoglycemia can occur as a rebound effect after high carbohydrate intake (known as the Somogyi phenomenon)
5. Irreversible brain damage and myocardial infarction can occur if hypoglycemia is not promptly corrected
6. Prompt reversal of hypoglycemia occurs with administration of concentrated glucose

B. Possible causes
1. Insulin overdose
2. Inadequate carbohydrate intake
3. Impaired glucose tolerance
4. Extrapancreatic tumor
5. Liver and adrenal insufficiency
6. Medical therapy, such as gastric surgery
7. Medications, such as sulfonylureas and beta blockers

C. Assessment findings
1. Cool, clammy skin
2. Headache
3. Diaphoresis
4. Dizziness
5. Staggering gait
6. Hunger
7. Nausea
8. Agitation
9. Fatigue
10. Anxiety
11. Tremors or seizures
12. Blurred vision
13. Inability to concentrate, progressing to alteration in LOC

D. Diagnostic test findings: serum glucose levels below 50 mg/dl

E. Patient care management
1. Goal: to elevate serum glucose levels promptly
2. Strategies

CLINICAL ALERT

a. Verify serum glucose level immediately by a fingerstick blood glucose method
(1) Serum glucose level must be verified immediately to determine if hypoglycemia is present
(2) Giving too much glucose can also injure the patient
(3) Delays in treating hypoglycemia must be avoided to prevent myocardial and neurologic tissue injury

b. Administer 50% glucose I.V. over 2 to 5 minutes if the patient is unconscious
c. Administer fluids I.V. for hydration and additional glucose for stabilization until oral intake is resumed
d. Give fast-acting carbohydrates, such as fruit juice, sugar, honey, and corn syrup, to relieve signs and symptoms if the patient is conscious
e. Follow with more complex carbohydrates, such as cheese and crackers, to stabilize serum glucose levels
f. Protect the patient from injury that may result from confusion, seizures, or coma
g. Teach the patient signs and symptoms of hypoglycemia and proper measures to correct it (for specific teaching tips, see *Recognizing hyperglycemia and hypoglycemia*)
h. Instruct the patient about the proper technique for blood glucose testing, and have the patient demonstrate the technique

TEACHING TIPS

Recognizing hyperglycemia and hypoglycemia

Be sure to include the following topics in your teaching plan for the patient with diabetes.

- Recognition of signs and symptoms of hyperglycemia
  - Dry, flushed skin
  - Nausea
  - Vomiting
  - Abdominal pain
  - Fever
  - Increased hunger
  - Increased thirst
  - Increased urine output
- Recognition of signs and symptoms of hypoglycemia
  - Cool, clammy skin
  - Headache
  - Sweating
  - Dizziness
  - Fatigue
  - Increased hunger
  - Increased thirst
  - Anxiety
  - Tremors

♦ VI. Syndrome of inappropriate antidiuretic hormone (SIADH)

A. General information
   1. SIADH is an endocrine dysfunction caused by uncontrolled production or excessive secretion of antidiuretic hormone (ADH)
   2. Normal ADH secretion is controlled by an increase in plasma osmolality, detection of decreased plasma volume in receptors located in the left atria and pulmonary vasculature, and detection of decreased blood pressure by carotid and aortic bodies
   3. Water is retained when ADH is secreted, and excessive secretion or production of ADH may result in water intoxication and cerebral edema
   4. As the kidneys attempt to compensate for the excess water, more sodium is filtered into the urine, causing severe hyponatremia

B. Causes
   1. Oat cell carcinoma of the lung
   2. Severe pneumonia
   3. Mechanical ventilation

4. Other cancers, such as leukemia and cancers of the pancreas, prostate, and brain
5. Head trauma
6. Stress
7. Medications, such as oral hypoglycemic agents, diuretics, and cytotoxic agents

C. Assessment findings
1. Weight gain without corresponding peripheral edema
2. Decreased and concentrated urine
3. Hypertension
4. Elevated CVP, PAP, PAWP
5. Nausea, vomiting, or diarrhea
6. Anorexia
7. Headache
8. Altered LOC
9. Seizures

D. Diagnostic test findings
1. Serum sodium level: less than 135 mEq/liter
2. Serum osmolality level: lower than urine osmolality level
3. Urine osmolality level: higher than serum osmolality level
4. Urine specific gravity: greater than 1.030
5. Plasma ADH level: elevated

E. Patient care management
1. Goals
   a. Correct cause
   b. Restore fluid and electrolyte balance
2. Strategies
   a. Assess the fluid balance carefully; monitor intake and output; restrict fluids based on amounts lost in urine and as insensible losses
   b. Replace sodium losses with I.V. administration of hypertonic 3% saline solution
   c. Administer diuretic therapy to promote water excretion
   d. Administer demeclocycline and lithium to inhibit the action of ADH on the renal tubules and to promote water excretion
   e. Prepare the patient for pulmonary artery catheter placement to monitor fluid status and evaluate therapy
   f. Assess and document CVP, PAP, PAWP, CO, and SVR
   g. Assess and document continuous ECG rhythm; vital signs; mental status; heart, lung, and bowel sounds; urine output; and any signs and symptoms indicating changes in these parameters
   h. Monitor urine and serum diagnostic tests for abnormalities; ensure laboratory specimens are obtained correctly and expedient-

ly so that an accurate correlation can be made between fluid and medication administration

i. Offer frequent mouth care and comfort measures when fluids are restricted
j. Weigh the patient daily at the same time and on the same scale with patient wearing the same amount of clothing to evaluate fluid balance
k. Prepare the patient for surgical intervention to remove the malignant lesion if it is the causative agent
l. Teach the patient the importance of fluid restriction and daily weighing

♦ VII. Diabetes insipidus (DI)

A. General information

1. DI is the physiologic reciprocal of SIADH
2. Decreased activity of ADH results in loss of free water from the body and profound dehydration and electrolyte disturbances
3. Two types of DI can occur
   a. Central (neurogenic) DI is more severe and accounts for 50% to 80% of all DI cases
   b. Renal (nephrogenic) DI is less severe and involves the reabsorption function of the kidneys
4. DI may be triphasic, especially after surgery
   a. Phase 1: transient occurrence lasting 2 to 3 days
   b. Phase 2: resolution
   c. Phase 3: recurrence after additional 2 to 3 days

B. Causes

1. Central DI
   a. Head injury
   b. Neurosurgery for tumor, aneurysm, or intracranial bleeding
   c. Meningitis or encephalitis
   d. Brain metastases, especially from leukemia or breast cancer
   e. Inherited defect of posterior pituitary gland
   f. Medications, including ethanol, reserpine, morphine, and phenytoin
2. Renal DI
   a. Polycystic kidney disease
   b. Pyelonephritis
   c. Pregnancy
   d. Inherited trait
   e. Medications, including lithium carbonate, demeclocycline, and methoxyflurane

C. Assessment findings
   1. Extreme polyuria, polydipsia, and nocturia
   2. Headache
   3. Fatigue and weakness
   4. Poor skin turgor and dry mucous membranes
   5. Tachycardia
   6. Postural hypotension
   7. Fever without diaphoresis
   8. Mental status changes, including lethargy, irritability, combativeness, and delirium

D. Diagnostic test findings
   1. Serum sodium level: greater than 150 mEq/L
   2. Serum osmolality level: higher than urine osmolality level
   3. Urine osmolality level: lower than serum osmolality level
   4. Urine specific gravity: less than 1.006
   5. Plasma ADH level: normal in renal DI; decreased in central DI

E. Patient care management
   1. Goals
      a. Correct cause
      b. Restore fluid and electrolyte balance
   2. Strategies
      a. Assess fluid balance carefully; monitor intake and output, including urine specific gravity; encourage oral fluid intake
      b. Administer I.V. fluids to correct dehydration
      c. Administer medications that enhance the action of ADH (for mild central DI), such as chlorpropamide, carbamazepine, and clofibrate
      d. Administer exogenous ADH (vasopressin) for severe central DI; may be given I.V., I.M., intranasally, or subcutaneously
      e. Administer thiazide diuretic with sodium-restricted diet for management of renal DI
      f. Prepare the patient for pulmonary artery catheter placement to monitor fluid status and evaluate therapy
      g. Assess and document CVP, PAP, PAWP, CO, and SVR
      h. Assess and document continuous ECG rhythm; vital signs; mental status; heart, lung, and bowel sounds; urine output; and signs and symptoms indicating changes in these parameters
      i. Monitor urine and serum diagnostic tests for abnormalities; ensure laboratory specimens are obtained correctly and expediently so that an accurate correlation can be made between fluid and medication administration
      j. Offer frequent mouth care and comfort measures when mucous membranes are dry

k. Assist body cooling by maintaining cool environment, cool drinks, tepid bath, light linens
l. Weigh the patient daily (at the same time on the same scale with the patient wearing the same amount of clothing) to evaluate fluid balance
m. Teach the patient the importance of daily weighing and adequate fluid intake to match fluid losses

♦ VIII. Thyrotoxicosis (thyroid storm or crisis)

A. General information
1. Thyrotoxicosis is a rapidly developing, life-threatening metabolic emergency caused by hyperthyroidism
2. Excessive thyroid hormone produces an increased rate of all metabolic processes
3. The mortality from thyrotoxicosis is greater than 20% if untreated

B. Causes
1. Graves' disease
2. Goiter or hyperfunctioning thyroid
3. Excessive intake of exogenous thyroid hormone
4. Abrupt cessation of antithyroid drugs
5. Trauma
6. Stress
7. Infection
8. DKA
9. Pregnancy-induced hypertension
10. Malignant tumor

C. Assessment findings
1. Heat intolerance
2. EXOPHTHALMOS or dryness of eyes
3. Enlarged thyroid gland
4. Hyperthermia
5. Dehydration
6. Diaphoresis
7. Flushing
8. Tachycardia and tachypnea
9. Nausea, vomiting, or diarrhea
10. Weight loss
11. Agitation or tremors

D. Diagnostic test findings
1. Triiodothyronine (T_3) and thyroxine (T_4) levels: elevated
2. Serum glucose level: increased (from glycogenolysis or decreased insulin production or secretion)
3. Serum calcium level: elevated (from increased bone metabolism)

4. Hb and HCT levels: elevated (from dehydration)
5. ECG: tachycardia even during sleep, with frequently occurring premature atrial and ventricular beats and, possibly, atrial fibrillation

E. Patient care management
1. Goals
   a. Support vital functions of the respiratory, cardiac, and renal systems
   b. Reverse peripheral effects of excessive thyroid hormone
2. Strategies
   a. Maintain a patent airway; ensure that the airway is not impaired by edema in the postoperative thyroidectomy patient
   b. Administer I.V. fluids for hydration and replacement of electrolytes
   c. Administer beta blockers to decrease the peripheral effects of thyroid hormone and to inhibit conversion of T_4 to T_3
   d. Administer propylthiouracil to inhibit conversion of T_4 to T_3
   e. Administer sodium or potassium iodide or Lugol's solution to inhibit release of iodine, which is essential for release of T_4 and T_3
   f. Administer glucocorticoids to block conversion of T_4 to T_3; this also may decrease adrenal insufficiency, which often accompanies thyrotoxicosis
   g. Administer drug therapy to treat the underlying disease, such as DKA
   h. Prepare the patient for pulmonary artery catheter placement to monitor fluid status and evaluate therapy
   i. Assess and document CVP, PAP, PAWP, CO, and SVR
   j. Assess and document continuous ECG rhythm; vital signs; mental status; heart, lung, and bowel sounds; urine output; and any signs and symptoms indicating changes in these parameters
   k. Maintain strict adherence to medication scheduling and dosing because drug conversion and degradation are increased
   l. Monitor T_3 and T_4 laboratory results, and report abnormal values
   m. Schedule activities to conserve the patient's energy
   n. Provide a quiet room to decrease stimuli and reduce metabolic demands
   o. Apply a cooling blanket for hyperthermia
   p. Provide safety measures to prevent accidental injury from altered LOC, seizures, or coma
   q. Avoid aspirin for fever control because it replaces T_3 from carrier protein and increases free T_3 levels
   r. Prepare the patient for surgical intervention to remove the malignant lesion if it is the causative agent
   s. Teach the patient the importance of hormonal replacement therapy and strict compliance

POINTS TO REMEMBER

- Fat breakdown for energy, in the absence of glucose, causes ketone formation.
- Irreversible brain damage and myocardial infarction can occur if hypoglycemia is not promptly reversed.
- When in doubt about glucose level, always give glucose; response will be immediate if the patient is hypoglycemic.
- Strict adherence to medication schedules and doses is imperative for patients with endocrine dysfunction who may have abnormal drug turnover and degradation because of alterations in metabolism.

STUDY QUESTIONS

To evaluate your understanding of this chapter, answer the following questions in the space provided; then compare your responses with the correct answers in Appendix B, pages 285 and 286.

1. Which metabolic functions are regulated by the secretion of hormones?
____
____

2. What might the nurse assess in a patient with DKA? ______________
____
____

3. What type of insulin and I.V. fluids are used initially to manage DKA? ___
____
____

4. Why does ketonemia not occur in HHNS? ______________
____
____

5. What is the initial management goal for hypoglycemia? ______________
____
____

6. What is the cause of SIADH? ______________________________

____

____

7. How do the kidneys compensate for excessive water retention that occurs in SIADH? ______________________________

____

____

8. What causes DI? ______________________________

____

____

9. Why is aspirin contraindicated for fever control in a thyrotoxicosis? ______

____

____

CRITICAL THINKING AND APPLICATION EXERCISES

1. Compare and contrast the clinical findings of DKA and HHNS. Present this information to a group of classmates.
2. Prepare drug information cards for the three most common types of insulin.
3. Demonstrate the use of a glucometer. Include skin preparation and infection-control practices.
4. Compare and contrast the clinical findings of SIADH and DI. Present this information to a group of classmates.
5. Prepare a diagram of the endocrine system. Include the organs and hormones, and describe the major functions of each.

CHAPTER

17

Neurologic Disorders

Learning objectives

After studying this chapter, you should be able to:

- Describe the general principles of neurologic function.
- Identify possible causes for each type of alteration in neurologic function.
- Discuss common assessment and diagnostic test findings for the patient with a specific alteration in neurologic function.
- Describe care management for the patient with a specific alteration in neurologic function.

Chapter overview

Caring for the patient with a neurologic disorder in an emergency or critical care area requires a sound understanding of the anatomy and physiology of the nervous system. Various causes contribute to each type of alteration in neurologic function. Common assessment and diagnostic test findings are used to determine the type and extent of dysfunction. Regardless of the cause, neurologic dysfunction creates the potential for significant deterioration in the body's function and the possibility of irreversible damage. Therefore, diagnosis and therapeutic interventions must be implemented in a timely manner to ensure quality of life after recovery. In general, care management for the patient with a specific alteration in neurologic dysfunction centers on supporting the patient's vital functions, treating the underlying cause of the dysfunction promptly, maintaining adequate cerebral blood flow, and minimizing the consequences of the dysfunction.

♦ I. Introduction

A. Functions
   1. The nervous system directs all movement, sensation, emotion, and thought by its control over all other body systems
   2. Any interruption in the nervous system or in its blood supply can produce life-threatening effects
   3. The extent of injury and the area of the brain involved determine the signs and symptoms exhibited

B. Risk factors
   1. Decreased blood flow to brain
   2. Trauma to head or spinal cord

C. Potential nursing diagnoses for the patient with a neurologic disorder
   1. Altered tissue perfusion
   2. Sensory or perceptual alterations
   3. Ineffective airway clearance
   4. Risk for injury
   5. Pain
   6. Self-care deficit
   7. Unilateral neglect
   8. Ineffective thermoregulation
   9. Impaired physical mobility
   10. Dysreflexia

♦ II. Anatomy and physiology

A. Central nervous system (CNS)
   1. The CNS consists of the brain, brain stem, and spinal cord
   2. The *cerebrum* has two hemispheres; specialized areas of each hemisphere perform motor, sensory, mental, and associative functions
   3. The *diencephalon* consists of the hypothalamus (which affects water balance, appetite, temperature, emotion, pituitary secretions, and autonomic functions) and the thalamus (which helps control primitive responses, such as fear and self-preservation, and acts as a relay point for most afferent and efferent tracts)
   4. The *cerebellum* coordinates muscle movement with sensory input, controls balance, and maintains muscle tone
   5. The *brain stem* consists of the midbrain, pons, and medulla oblongata; it relays messages between the brain and the lower levels of the nervous system

6. Four *communicating ventricles* contain cerebrospinal fluid (CSF) and include two lateral ventricles and a third and fourth ventricle
7. The *spinal cord* mediates the reflex arc and is the communicating pathway between the brain and the peripheral nervous system
8. The brain receives approximately 20% of cardiac output, which provides a constant supply of oxygen and glucose to the brain cells

B. Peripheral nervous system
1. The peripheral nervous system consists of the cranial and spinal nerves
2. The 12 pairs of cranial nerves primarily serve the motor and sensory needs of the head as well as those of the neck, chest, and abdomen
3. The 31 pairs of spinal nerves include 8 cervical, 12 thoracic, 5 lumbar, 5 sacral, and 1 coccygeal; they supply the upper and lower extremities

C. Compensatory mechanisms
1. Sufficient cerebral blood flow is necessary to meet the metabolic needs of the brain and depends on an intact cerebrovascular system
2. Two compensatory mechanisms protect the brain under adverse conditions
   a. Collateral circulation allows for alternate blood flow if normal blood flow is occluded
   b. Autoregulation maintains constant blood flow through vasodilation or constriction stimulated by serum carbon dioxide and oxygen concentration and arterial blood pressure; autoregulation fails to function with mean arterial pressure less than 60 mm Hg or pathology associated with atherosclerosis, arterial rupture, or occlusion

♦ III. Cerebrovascular accident (CVA)

A. General information
1. CVA is a sudden, severe disruption of the blood supply to the brain, producing cerebral anoxia and alteration in cerebral metabolism
2. CVA is classified as thrombotic or hemorrhagic
   a. *Thrombotic CVA* occurs when a cerebral artery is occluded by a thrombus or an embolus
   b. *Hemorrhagic CVA* occurs from an intracerebral hemorrhage (ICH) or subarachnoid hemorrhage (SAH)
3. CVA may also be categorized according to the side of the brain affected, either right or left
4. The signs and symptoms vary, depending on the side of the brain affected

B. Causes
1. Thrombus
2. Cerebral embolism
3. Ruptured intracerebral artery, commonly from hypertension (ICH)
4. Ruptured aneurysm or ruptured arteriovenous malformation (SAH)

C. Assessment findings
1. Left CVA
   a. Right hemiparesis or hemiplegia
   b. Right homonymous hemianopia (unilateral impaired vision, visual field cuts)
   c. Memory deficits in language
   d. Expressive or receptive aphasia
   e. Slow, cautious behavior
   f. Acute intellectual impairment
2. Right CVA
   a. Left hemiparesis or hemiplegia
   b. Left homonymous hemianopia
   c. Memory deficits in performance
   d. Impulsive behavior
   e. Lack of motivation
   f. Spatial and perceptual deficits

D. Diagnostic test findings
1. Computed tomographic (CT) scan: identifies the location and characteristics of a CVA or the distortion or shift of ventricles with hemorrhage or edema
2. Magnetic resonance imaging: identifies changes in the cranial and spinal structures
3. EEG: identifies seizure activity and changes in the brain's electrical waveforms
4. Angiography: identifies occlusion, stenosis, aneurysms, hemorrhage, and infarction of the arterial system

E. Patient care management
1. Goals
   a. Support vital functions
   b. Restore cerebral blood flow
   c. Minimize neurologic deficits
   d. Prevent progression
2. Strategies
   a. Maintain a patent airway to promote adequate oxygenation
   b. Administer oxygen therapy with possible intubation and mechanical ventilation to ensure adequate tissue perfusion
   c. Maintain bed rest to minimize metabolic requirements

d. Provide I.V. fluids to support blood pressure and maintain volume
e. Administer dexamethasone to reduce cerebral edema
f. Administer anticoagulants and antiplatelet drugs for thrombotic conditions after hemorrhage has been ruled out
g. Administer sedatives, such as phenobarbital, to decrease metabolic requirements
h. Assess the patient's neurologic status; observe for CVA progression and level of consciousness (LOC) changes as evidenced by decreasing numerical score on the GLASGOW COMA SCALE (see *Assessing level of consciousness using the Glasgow coma scale,* page 192)
i. Correct cardiovascular abnormalities, such as atrial fibrillation, that may be contributing factors
j. Consider surgical procedures to correct circulatory impairment, prevent repeated hemorrhage, or relieve cerebral pressure
k. Begin bedside range-of-motion exercises to preserve mobility and prevent deformities
l. Teach the patient to identify risk factors and necessary lifestyle modifications, such as diet, stress reduction, and smoking cessation
m. Direct the family to community groups that provide support or rehabilitation

♦ IV. Meningitis

A. General information
1. Meningitis is an inflammation of the brain and spinal cord that may involve all meningeal membranes
2. Meningitis is classified as bacterial, fungal, or viral
   a. *Bacterial meningitis* is commonly a complication of bacteremia
   b. *Fungal meningitis* is caused by fungal infections of the CNS
   c. *Viral meningitis* occurs as a complication of systemic viral infections
3. The most common type of meningitis is bacterial, a medical emergency that may be fatal within a few days if not treated
4. Prompt recognition of the causative organism ensures the best prognosis
5. Permanent secondary damage and death can occur from the cerebral edema associated with the inflammation
6. Prevalence of meningitis increases in people who live in crowded conditions and those in contact with farm animals, ticks, or fleas

Assessing level of consciousness using the Glasgow coma scale

To assess a patient's level of consciousness quickly in an emergency, use the Glasgow coma scale. The chart below is an expanded version of this useful — though not comprehensive — assessment technique. (A patient scoring 7 or lower is comatose and probably has severe neurologic damage.)

TEST	SCORE	PATIENT'S RESPONSE
Verbal response (when you ask: "What year is this?")		
Oriented	5	Tells you the current year
Confused	4	Tells you an incorrect year
Inappropriate words	3	Replies randomly (for example, "roses")
Incomprehensible	2	Moans or screams
None	1	Gives no response
Eye opening response		
Spontaneously	4	Opens eyes spontaneously
To speech	3	Opens eyes when asked
To pain	2	Opens eyes only on painful stimulus (for example, application of pressure to bony ridge under eyebrow)
None	1	Doesn't open eyes in response to any stimulus
Motor response		
Obeys commands	6	Shows two fingers when asked
Localizes pain	5	Reaches toward the painful stimulation and tries to remove it or push it away
Withdraws	4	Moves away from a painful stimulus
Abnormal flexion	3	Assumes a decorticate posture (below) 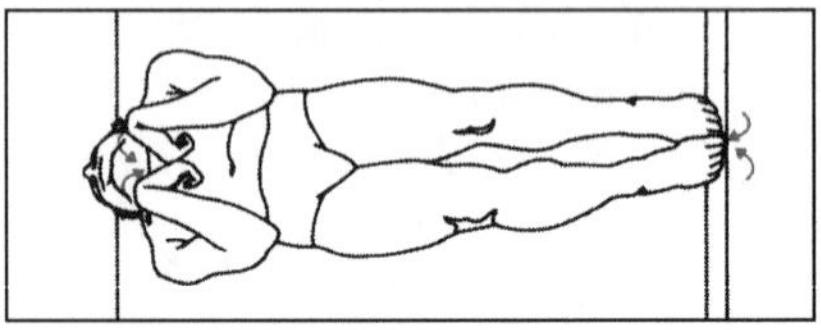
Abnormal extension	2	Assumes a decerebrate posture (below) 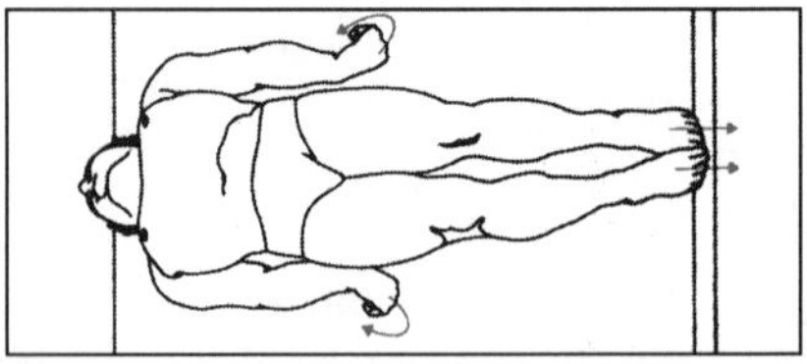
None	1	Doesn't respond; just lies flaccid — an ominous sign

B. Causes
1. Bacterial meningitis
   a. Otitis media
   b. Respiratory infection or sinusitis
   c. Bacteremia
   d. Immunologic reactions
   e. Metastatic infections
2. Fungal meningitis
   a. Complication of acquired immunodeficiency syndrome
   b. Histoplasmosis
   c. Contaminated needles or syringes from drug abuse
3. Viral meningitis
   a. Enteroviruses
   b. Mumps
   c. Herpes simplex
   d. Chickenpox
   e. Arbovirus

C. Assessment findings
1. Bacterial meningitis
   a. Nuchal rigidity
   b. Chills
   c. Fever
   d. Lethargy
   e. Positive BRUDZINSKI'S SIGN and KERNIG'S SIGN
   f. Nausea and vomiting
   g. Headache
   h. Generalized seizures
2. Fungal meningitis
   a. Headache
   b. Fever
   c. Personality changes
   d. Positive Brudzinski's and Kernig's signs
3. Viral meningitis
   a. Headache
   b. Pain when moving the eyes
   c. Weakness
   d. Painful extremities
   e. Positive Brudzinski's and Kernig's signs

D. Diagnostic test findings
1. Lumbar puncture: identifies the type of causative agent by abnormality of glucose, protein, and white blood cell (WBC) count
2. Blood cultures: positive for causative organism

(Text continues on page 196.)

DECISION TREE

Nursing care in meningitis

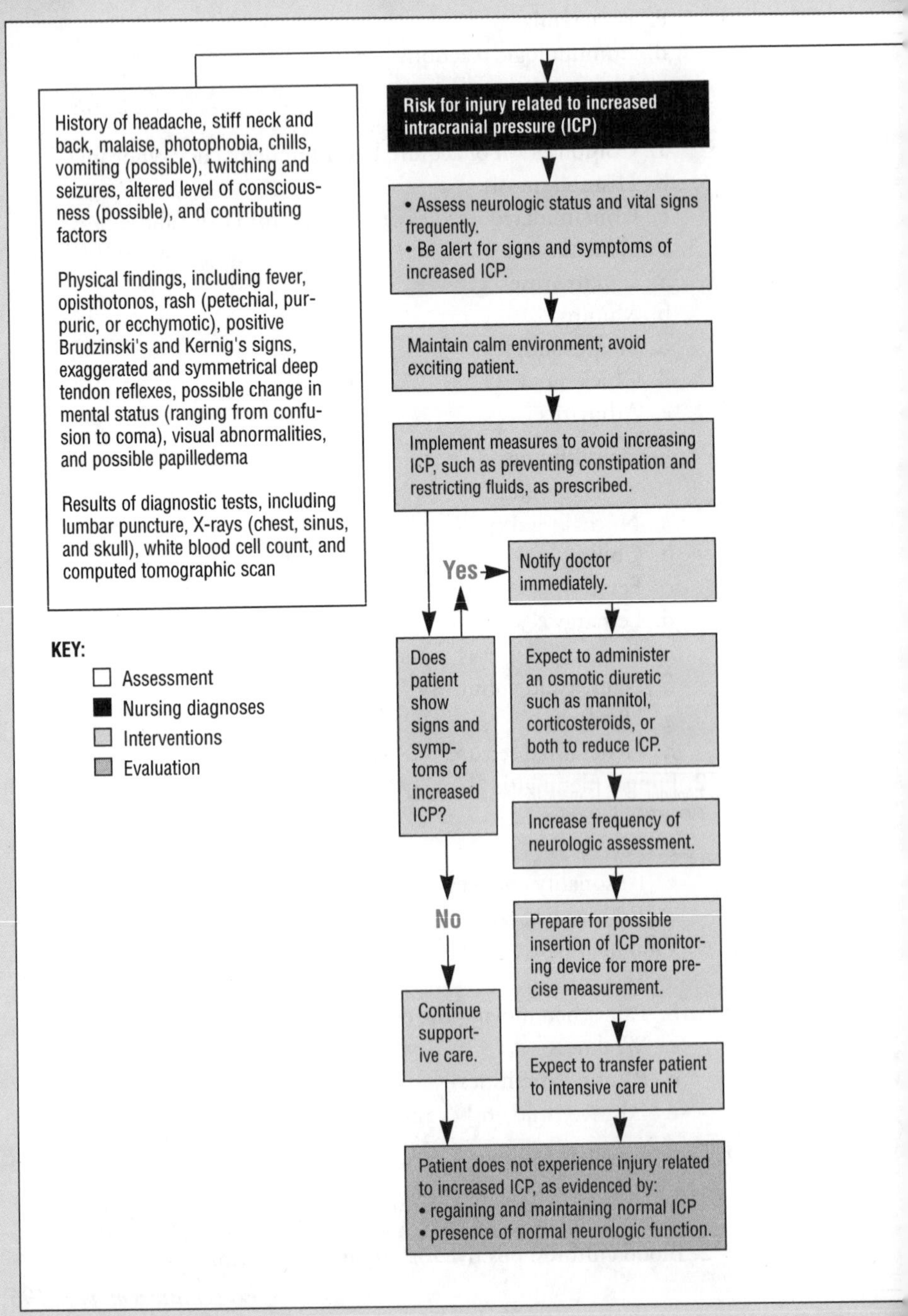

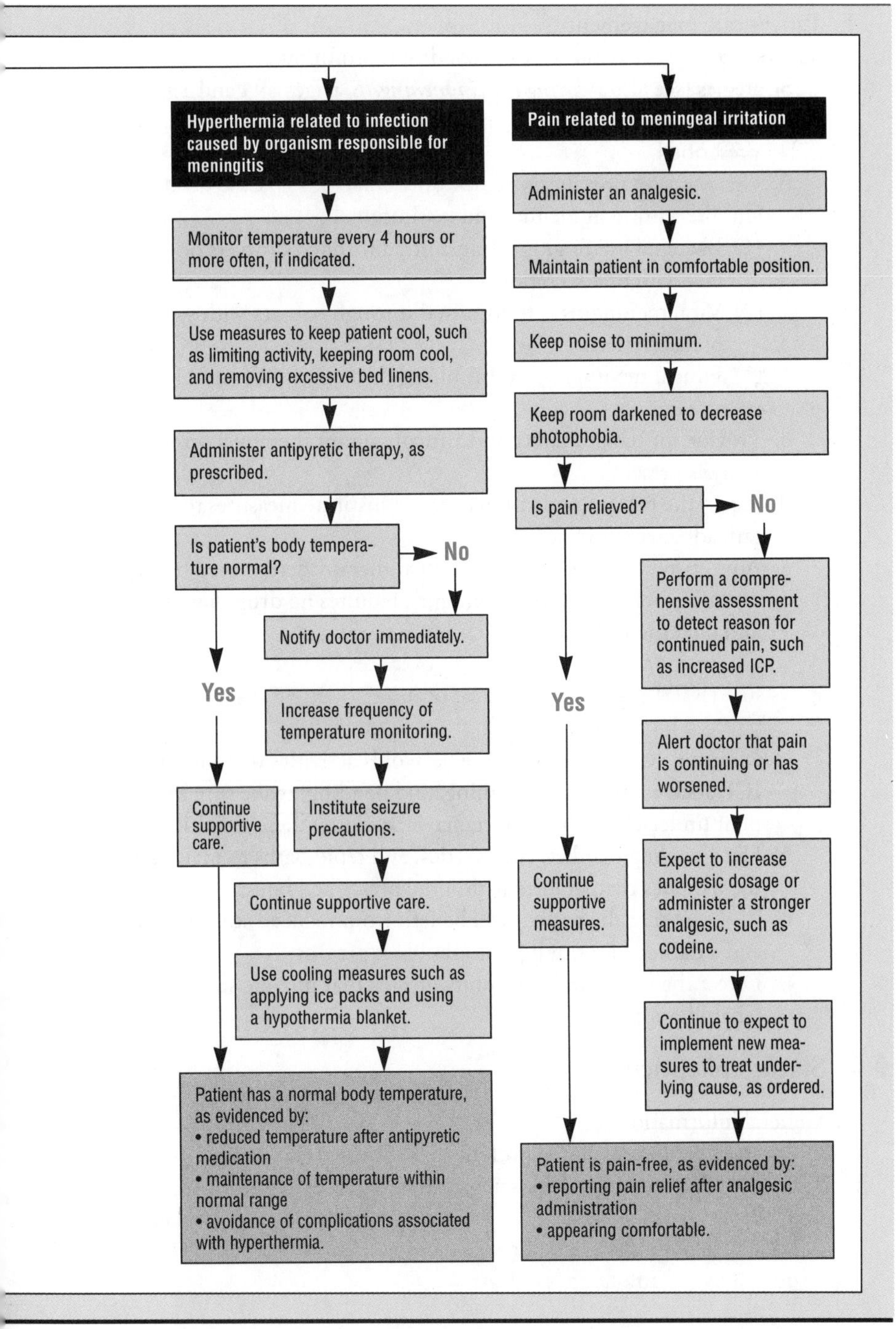
Hyperthermia related to infection caused by organism responsible for meningitis
Monitor temperature every 4 hours or more often, if indicated.
Use measures to keep patient cool, such as limiting activity, keeping room cool, and removing excessive bed linens.
Administer antipyretic therapy, as prescribed.
Is patient's body temperature normal?
No
Notify doctor immediately.
Increase frequency of temperature monitoring.
Institute seizure precautions.
Continue supportive care.
Use cooling measures such as applying ice packs and using a hypothermia blanket.
Yes
Continue supportive care.
Patient has a normal body temperature, as evidenced by:
• reduced temperature after antipyretic medication
• maintenance of temperature within normal range
• avoidance of complications associated with hyperthermia.
Pain related to meningeal irritation
Administer an analgesic.
Maintain patient in comfortable position.
Keep noise to minimum.
Keep room darkened to decrease photophobia.
Is pain relieved?
No
Perform a comprehensive assessment to detect reason for continued pain, such as increased ICP.
Alert doctor that pain is continuing or has worsened.
Expect to increase analgesic dosage or administer a stronger analgesic, such as codeine.
Continue to expect to implement new measures to treat underlying cause, as ordered.
Yes
Continue supportive measures.
Patient is pain-free, as evidenced by:
• reporting pain relief after analgesic administration
• appearing comfortable.

3. Counter immunoelectrophoresis: bacterial antigens in CSF and urine
4. WBC count: elevated in presence of infection

E. Patient care management
1. Goal: to diagnose and treat the condition promptly
2. Strategies (see also *Nursing care in meningitis,* pages 194 and 195)
    a. Maintain a patent airway and provide supplemental oxygen, as prescribed
    b. Use isolation precautions based on Centers for Disease Control and Prevention guidelines and institutional policy
        (1) Bacterial meningitis is transmitted through droplets or contact with oral secretions
        (2) Viral meningitis is transmitted through contact with stool or oral secretions
        (3) Fungal meningitis is transmitted through the air and bloodstream
    c. Provide for patient safety and anticonvulsant therapy if seizure activity is present
    d. Assess the patient's nutritional status; institute measures to maintain adequate nutrition
    e. Administer antibiotic and antifungal therapy determined by the causative organism (viral meningitis requires no drug therapy), and document the patient's response to therapy

CLINICAL ALERT

    f. Observe for signs and symptoms of increased intracranial pressure (ICP), such as headaches, vomiting, fluctuations in heart rate and blood pressure, and widening pulse pressure
    g. Monitor the patient to be sure he avoids activities that increase ICP, such as straining, coughing, and bending; make sure the patient understands the importance of avoiding these activities
    h. Use a cooling blanket, antipyretics, and tepid baths to maintain the patient's temperature within the prescribed range
    i. Be aware that the patient will benefit from reduced stimulation and a darkened room if photophobia is present
    j. Direct the family to community groups that provide support or rehabilitation

♦ V. Status epilepticus

A. General information
1. Status epilepticus is acute, prolonged seizure activity that occurs without full recovery of consciousness between convulsions
2. Status epilepticus is a medical emergency because the constant activity may deplete the brain of oxygen and glucose, which may produce hypoxia and neuronal death

B. Causes

1. Noncompliance with medication treatment
2. Concurrent infection
3. Alcohol abuse
4. Fever

C. Assessment findings

1. Alteration in LOC
2. Tonic or clonic body movements
3. Incontinence of urine or stool
4. Automatisms: involuntary motor activities, such as lip smacking, swallowing, and chewing

D. Diagnostic test findings

1. Serum chemistries: metabolic or electrolyte imbalance
2. Serum alcohol level: positive for presence and quantity of alcohol
3. EEG: negative for other pathological conditions
4. CT scan: negative for other pathological conditions
5. Anticonvulsant serum drug levels: subtherapeutic or therapeutic amount of drug in blood

E. Patient care management

1. Goals
   a. Ensure adequate cerebral oxygenation
   b. Stop seizure activity
2. Strategies
   a. Maintain a patent airway and adequate oxygenation, with possible intubation
   b. Administer short-term anticonvulsant therapy, such as diazepam or lorazepam, until the patient is seizure-free
   c. Administer long-acting anticonvulsant therapy, such as phenytoin or phenobarbital; infuse phenytoin I.V. with normal saline solution only to avoid a reaction with dextrose-containing solutions
   d. Consider general anesthesia or neuromuscular blocking agents to stop seizure activity if other anticonvulsants are unsuccessful
   e. Protect the patient during seizure activity: avoid restraining the patient or forcing anything through clenched teeth; move potentially dangerous items away from the patient
   f. Keep the patient turned to the side during the seizure to prevent aspiration
   g. Monitor and document duration of seizure activity, associated signs, and the patient's LOC after seizure activity
   h. Reassure and reorient the patient when he awakens to alleviate anxiety

TEACHING TIPS

Patient with a seizure disorder

Be sure to include the following topics in your teaching plan for a patient with a seizure disorder.

- Signs and symptoms necessitating medical attention
- Importance of complying with treatment
- Management of the patient during a seizure episode
- Activation of the emergency medical system, if needed
- Importance of having the patient wear a medical identification bracelet
- Medication regimen, including dosage, scheduling, and adverse effects
- Avoidance of caffeine and other drugs that can precipitate seizure activity
- Gum care while on antiseizure medications, especially phenytoin
- Necessary lifestyle changes, such as restriction against driving motor vehicles, operating heavy equipment, or swimming until the patient is seizure-free for a specified time

i. Document the name of the drug, the last dose, and the medication regimen if the patient is taking anticonvulsant medications

j. Teach the patient and family about all aspects of the disorder and its management (for specific teaching tips, see *Patient with a seizure disorder*)

♦ VI. Myasthenic crisis

A. General information

1. Myasthenic crisis is the sudden onset of weakness often manifested by sudden respiratory distress or the inability to speak or swallow
2. Myasthenia gravis is an autoimmune disease in which antibodies attack the acetylcholine receptor sites at the postsynaptic membrane, impairing neuromuscular transmission
3. Progressive weakness of the diaphragm and intercostal muscles is a medical emergency because it may lead to respiratory failure
4. The patient with myasthenia gravis may develop other crises in response to drug therapy
   a. *Cholinergic crisis* may occur from overmedication with anticholinesterase drugs
   b. *Brittle crisis* may occur from desensitivity of receptors at the neuromuscular junction to anticholinesterase drugs
5. The patient with myasthenia gravis should recognize the risk factors that precipitate myasthenic crisis, such as emotional stress, systemic infections, and exposure to heat or cold

B. Causes
  1. Progression of the disease
  2. Systemic infections
  3. Emotional stress
  4. Surgery
  5. Trauma
  6. Certain drugs, such as morphine, beta blockers, some anticonvulsants, cardiac drugs, and antibiotics
  7. Exposure to heat or cold

C. Assessment findings
  1. Decrease in chest expansion and air movement
  2. Weakness of the ocular, respiratory, and bulbar muscles
  3. Increased anxiety
  4. Dysphagia
  5. DYSARTHRIA
  6. PTOSIS
  7. Diplopia

D. Diagnostic test findings: signs and symptoms may be so significant for myasthenia gravis that diagnosis may be made on the basis of history and physical examination
  1. Tensilon test: muscle weakness and fatigue decrease within 1 minute; the improvement lasts for up to 5 minutes after I.V. administration of edrophonium chloride (Tensilon)
  2. Neostigmine bromide test: muscle weakness and fatigue improve within 15 minutes and last for up to 2 hours after I.M. administration of neostigmine
  3. Electromyography: rapid decrease in the amplitude of evoked potentials
  4. Serum antibodies against acetylcholine receptor: positive

E. Patient care management
  1. Goals
     a. Provide respiratory support
     b. Preserve remaining muscle function
     c. Reduce and remove circulating antibodies
  2. Strategies
     a. Maintain a patent airway, provide supplemental oxygen, and consider mechanical respiratory support, if necessary
     b. Administer anticholinesterase drugs, such as neostigmine, to increase the availability of acetylcholine at the neuromuscular junction
     c. Begin immunosuppressive therapy, such as administering corticosteroids, using plasmapheresis, or preparing for thymectomy

CLINICAL ALERT

d. Assess the patient for the presence of a gag reflex and the ability to swallow
e. Administer medications at the exact times ordered; delay in administration time may result in difficulty in swallowing
f. Place the patient in a sitting position with the neck slightly flexed to aid swallowing
g. Determine effective ways to communicate with the patient so his needs are met
h. Administer artificial tears to protect corneas in the patient with ptosis
i. Teach the patient and family the importance of taking medications at the prescribed times; be sure they know risk factors and can recognize signs and symptoms warranting medical attention, such as respiratory distress, ptosis, diplopia, and dysphasia

♦ VII. Increased intracranial pressure (ICP)

A. General information

1. ICP is an elevation of the pressure exerted within the skull by intracranial volume above 15 mm Hg
2. Increased ICP is not a disease but the result of conditions that alter intracranial volume
3. When ICP increases to pathological levels, brain damage can occur because the rigid skull allows little space for expansion
4. The contents of the intracranial vault includes the brain, CSF, and cerebral blood flow
5. The brain compensates for increases in ICP by regulating the intracranial volume (limiting blood flow to the head), displacing CSF into the spinal canal, and increasing or decreasing CSF production
6. When compensatory mechanisms become overworked, small changes in intracranial volume lead to large changes in ICP
7. Hypercapnia and hypoxia contribute to changes in ICP because they cause cerebral vasodilation, which in turn increases blood volume and ICP

B. Causes

1. Head injuries
2. Aneurysms
3. CVA
4. Brain tumors
5. Reye's syndrome
6. Impaired autoregulation
7. Hydrocephalus

C. Assessment findings
1. Deteriorating LOC
2. Pupillary dilation
3. Decreased pupillary light reflex
4. Loss of motor function
5. Sensory deterioration
6. Vital sign changes
7. Vomiting

D. Diagnostic test findings
1. CT scan: cerebral structure shifts from tumor, hematomas, or hydrocephalus
2. Brain scan: cerebral hemorrhage, hematoma, or tumor
3. ICP monitoring: increased ICP

E. Patient care management
1. Goals
   a. Reduce ICP
   b. Improve cerebral perfusion pressure (CPP)
   c. Decrease brain tissue distortion
2. Strategies
   a. Maintain a patent airway; intubate and mechanically ventilate to prevent hypoxia and hypercapnia
   b. Consider surgery to remove intracranial masses
   c. Administer osmotic agents, such as mannitol and urea, to decrease CSF volume and increase CPP (use is controversial because of cerebral edema)
   d. Consider diuretics, such as furosemide, to decrease CSF volume
   e. Administer steroids, such as dexamethasone, to reduce brain edema and ICP
   f. Drain CSF if a ventricular drainage system is in place, based on the doctor's order and the patient's condition
   g. Consider administering drugs such as propranolol in combination with neuromuscular blockers to decrease cerebral oxygen demand
   h. Use the Glasgow coma scale and the institution's neurologic flow sheet to assess changes in LOC
   i. Monitor ABG measurements to prevent hypoxia and hypercapnia
   j. Maintain partial pressures of carbon dioxide in arterial blood between 30 and 35 mm Hg to prevent cerebral vasodilation produced by hypercapnia
   k. Keep partial pressures of oxygen in arterial blood within normal limits to prevent cerebral vasodilation produced by hypoxia

l. Preoxygenate and ventilate before and after suctioning to prevent hypoxia; consider administering lidocaine to reduce spasm of airway before suctioning

m. Limit suctioning to 15 seconds to prevent hypoxia

CLINICAL ALERT

n. Elevate the head of the bed 15 to 30 degrees or as ordered to facilitate venous return

o. Know that the head of the bed can be kept flat to improve cerebral bloodflow with only a minimal elevation of ICP

p. Avoid neck rotation, flexion, or extension to facilitate venous return

q. If a tracheostomy or endotracheal tube is required, make sure ties are not too tight to impede venous return

r. Space out activities known to increase ICP, such as suctioning, turning, and Valsalva's maneuver

♦ VIII. Autonomic dysreflexia (AD)

A. General information

1. AD may occur in patients with spinal cord injuries at the T-6 level or above after spinal shock has resolved
2. It is characterized by an uninhibited sympathetic nervous system response occurring below the level of the spinal cord lesion caused by lack of control from higher centers, producing uncontrolled, rapidly occurring hypertension
3. AD is classified as a medical emergency because the resultant hypertension may produce life-threatening consequences, such as seizures, CVA, and SAH

CLINICAL ALERT

4. It is caused by a variety of stimuli, including nursing interventions aimed at the preventive aspects of care
5. Although AD occurs most frequently during the first year after a spinal cord injury, it is considered a lifelong problem

B. Causes

1. Distended bladder from urine retention
2. Kinking or blockage of indwelling (Foley) catheter, if in place
3. Genitourinary infection
4. Fecal impaction
5. Pressure ulcer
6. Uterine contractions during labor
7. Drafts in room

C. Assessment findings

1. Hypertension
2. Severe headache
3. Bradycardia or tachycardia
4. Pallor and coolness below the level of the lesion

5. Flushing and sweating above the level of the lesion
6. Nasal stuffiness
7. Blurred vision
8. Pilomotor erection

D. Diagnostic test findings
1. Hypertension is the primary finding
2. Blood pressure readings commonly reach 240 to 300 mm Hg systolic and 150 mm Hg diastolic

E. Patient care management
1. Goals
   a. Determine and remove the causative stimulus, if possible
   b. Minimize complications resulting from the disorder
2. Strategies
   a. Elevate the head of the bed or place the patient in a sitting position to promote cerebral venous return
   b. Monitor blood pressure and heart rate and rhythm
   c. Notify the doctor if symptoms do not resolve, particularly severe hypertension
   d. Recognize factors that may precipitate AD, such as bladder distention and fecal impaction, and institute measures to prevent or correct them
   e. Recognize that ganglionic blocking agents, such as hydralazine hydrochloride (Apresoline), may be required to block hyperreflexia
   f. Maintain a calm and reassuring manner during the acute episode, recognizing that stress increases sympathetic response
   g. Provide patient and family teaching after the acute episode has resolved; review signs and symptoms, prevention methods, and treatments

POINTS TO REMEMBER

- Autoregulation is maintained in the brain by vasodilation or constriction and serum oxygen and carbon dioxide levels.
- The Glasgow coma scale is an objective way to measure LOC.
- Bacterial meningitis is the most common type of meningitis.
- Signs of meningeal irritation include nuchal rigidity and positive Brudzinski's and Kernig's signs.
- The best treatment of autonomic dysreflexia is prevention.

Study questions

To evaluate your understanding of this chapter, answer the following questions in the space provided; then compare your responses with the correct answers in Appendix B, page 286.

1. Which two compensatory mechanisms protect the brain under adverse conditions? ______________________________

____

____

2. How do assessment findings differ in left CVA and right CVA? __________

____

____

3. What is the key diagnostic test for meningitis? ______________________________

____

____

4. How does the brain compensate for increases in ICP? ______________

____

____

Critical thinking and application exercises

1. Develop a chart describing the interventions a nurse would use to determine the cause of an episode of autonomic dysreflexia.
2. Follow a patient with a CVA from admission through discharge. Develop a plan of care, including any need for follow-up and home care.
3. Develop a presentation for your classmates describing the major drugs used to treat increased ICP and the rationale behind each.
4. List two strategies that can be used to enhance safety in a patient with homonymous hemianopia.

CHAPTER

18

Gastrointestinal Disorders

Learning objectives

After studying this chapter, you should be able to:

- Describe the general principles of GI system function.
- Identify possible causes for each type of alteration in GI function.
- Discuss common assessment and diagnostic test findings for the patient with a specific GI disorder.
- Describe care management for the patient with a specific alteration in GI function.

Chapter overview

Caring for the patient with a GI disorder requires an understanding of GI anatomy and physiology. A thorough assessment is essential to planning and implementing care. The assessment includes a history, identification of causes and risk factors, examination for signs and symptoms, and diagnostic test findings. Nursing diagnoses focus primarily on alteration in nutrition, fluid volume deficits, alteration in bowel function, alteration in tissue perfusion, pain, and anxiety. The major goals of patient care management are to correct the causative factors, prevent further damage and complications, control bleeding, maintain fluid volume status, and relieve pain and anxiety.

♦ I. Introduction

A. Structure and function
   1. The GI system, which is also called the alimentary tract or the digestive system, begins at the mouth and ends at the anus
   2. The GI system functions to mechanically and chemically alter ingested food so that nutritional needs are met

B. Risk factors
   1. Alcohol
   2. Drugs, such as aspirin and nonsteroidal anti-inflammatory drugs
   3. Smoking
   4. Stress and trauma
   5. Infection

C. Potential nursing diagnoses for the patient with GI dysfunction
   1. Altered nutrition: less than body requirements
   2. Fluid volume deficit
   3. Constipation
   4. Diarrhea
   5. Altered tissue perfusion
   6. Anxiety
   7. Pain

♦ II. Anatomy and physiology

A. Structures
   1. The GI system consists of the mouth, esophagus, stomach, small intestine, and large intestine
   2. Four accessory organs aid the digestive system: salivary glands, pancreas, gallbladder, and liver

B. Blood supply
   1. The arterial blood supply to the GI tract is primarily delivered through the mesenteric arteries
   2. The portal venous system collects and delivers venous blood from the GI tract to the liver and back into the inferior vena cava

C. Regulation: under control of the autonomic nervous system

♦ III. Bleeding esophageal varices

A. General information
   1. Bleeding esophageal varices are varicose veins in the esophagus that have ruptured; they most commonly occur in the distal esophagus
   2. Portal hypertension with pressures elevated from the normal 8 to 12 mm Hg to more than 30 mm Hg causes hypertrophy of veins and risk of rupture

3. The mortality rate from bleeding esophageal varices may be as high as 60% with the first episode
4. Rebleeding, with a higher mortality rate, is likely within the first year

B. Causes
1. Cirrhosis
2. Hepatitis
3. Biliary infection or biliary disease, including stones or tumor
4. Trauma, including surgery to portal venous system

C. Assessment findings
1. Sudden and painless hematemesis
2. Hypovolemia from blood loss
3. MELENA
4. Other signs and symptoms of GI bleeding or hepatic failure (see "Acute GI bleeding: Ulcer," pages 208 to 210, and "Hepatic failure," pages 216 to 218)

D. Diagnostic test findings
1. Complete blood count (CBC): decreased hemoglobin (Hb) and hematocrit (HCT) levels and platelet count
2. Liver enzyme levels (lactate dehydrogenase, serum alanine aminotransferase, serum aspartate aminotransferase): elevated
3. Blood urea nitrogen (BUN): increased level
4. Prothrombin time (PT): prolonged
5. Endoscopy: visualizes and localizes source of bleeding

E. Patient care management
1. Goals
   a. Control the bleeding
   b. Prevent complications of shock and further liver failure
2. Strategies
   a. Administer oxygen if hypoxia is present; monitor SaO_2 with pulse oximeter
   b. Intubate and mechanically ventilate if the patient cannot maintain breathing
   c. Administer vasopressin to constrict mesenteric, splenic, and hepatic arterioles and to decrease blood flow to portal system
   d. Administer nitroprusside or nitroglycerin, if required, to decrease peripheral vasoconstriction
   e. Prepare the patient for BALLOON TAMPONADE with such devices as a Sengstaken-Blakemore, Minnesota, or Linton tube to temporarily control bleeding

f. Maintain balloon tamponade by using adequate pressure inflation and deflation with traction to maintain position, as ordered, to prevent tissue necrosis from excessive pressure

CLINICAL ALERT

g. Do not release pressure on the gastric balloon before the esophageal balloon is deflated because this can cause the balloon to rise in the oropharynx and occlude the airway; keep scissors at the bedside for prompt cutting and removal of balloon tamponade if gastric balloon ruptures
h. Suction patient as needed to remove oral secretions that cannot be swallowed when the esophageal balloon is inflated
i. Administer I.V. fluids for hydration and volume expansion to replace losses; avoid using saline solutions, except with blood products, which contribute to ascites and edema
j. Administer blood products, according to institution's protocol, to replace losses and maintain HCT count
k. Prepare the patient for pulmonary artery catheter placement to monitor fluid status and evaluate therapy
l. Assess and document central venous pressure (CVP), pulmonary artery pressure (PAP), pulmonary artery wedge pressure (PAWP), cardiac output (CO), and systemic vascular resistance (SVR)
m. Assess and document continuous electrocardiogram (ECG) rhythm; vital signs; mental status; heart, lung, and bowel sounds; urine output; and any signs and symptoms indicating changes in these parameters
n. Prepare the patient for sclerotherapy (dilated varices are injected with a sclerosing agent, causing fibrosis) to control bleeding
o. Monitor Hb and HCT levels, and report abnormal results
p. Measure and record losses from bleeding
q. Administer parenteral nutrition to support the patient's metabolic needs and defend against infection
r. Prevent transmission of infection by washing hands thoroughly and wearing gloves if contact with blood or body fluids is likely
s. Offer frequent mouth care and comfort measures when fluids are restricted
t. Provide emotional support to decrease fear and anxiety
u. Prepare the patient for possible implantation of a portacaval shunt to reduce portal hypertension

♦ IV. Acute GI bleeding: Ulcer

A. General information

1. Acute GI bleeding is a life-threatening emergency caused by ulceration of the GI mucosa and characterized by gross vomiting or defecation of occult stool

2. Upper GI hemorrhage is produced from any site proximal to the cecum and includes ulcers of the mouth, stomach, or duodenum as well as gastritis and esophageal varices
3. Peptic ulcer disease includes duodenal and gastric ulcers
4. Most ulcers are duodenal and occur during middle age
5. Gastric ulcers occurring after age 50 are likely to become malignant
6. Lower GI hemorrhage is produced from any site distal to the cecum and includes ruptured diverticula and ischemic bowel polyps, tumors, and eroding aortic aneurysm
7. Ulcerative erosion occurs from excess hydrochloric acid (HCl)
8. Most acute GI bleeding is from an arterial source
9. Estimated blood loss is an index to the severity of the bleeding
10. Blood loss greater than 20% causes decreased venous return and CO

B. Causes
1. Stress
2. Trauma, including surgery
3. Burns
4. Drugs that stimulate HCl release, such as reserpine; those that decrease blood supply to the GI tract, such as vasopressors; and those that alter mucosal integrity, such as aspirin, anticoagulants, and steroids
5. Stimulants, such as nicotine and caffeine
6. Biliary or pancreatic disease

C. Assessment findings
1. Hematemesis
2. Melena (black, tarlike stool)
3. Hematochezia (bloody stool)
4. Diarrhea
5. Mild to severe abdominal pain
6. Weakness
7. Dysphagia or heartburn
8. Signs of shock, including hypotension, tachycardia, diaphoresis, pallor, and decreased urine output

D. Diagnostic test findings
1. Stool GUAIAC TEST: positive
2. Emesis guaiac test: positive
3. Hb and HCT tests: decreased levels
4. Arterial blood gas (ABG) measurements: acidosis if shock is present, causing lactic acidosis
5. ECG: ischemic changes if hypoperfusion exists
6. Endoscopy: source of the bleeding visualized and localized
7. Biopsy: if cancer is the source of the bleeding
8. Upper and lower GI tract X-rays: air and contrast (barium) indicating area of bleeding

E. Patient care management
  1. Goal: to control shock and bleeding
  2. Strategies
    a. Maintain a patent airway to prevent aspiration of emesis or blood
    b. Administer oxygen therapy to treat hypoxia from a decrease in Hb levels; monitor SaO_2 with pulse oximeter
    c. Administer I.V. fluids, both crystalloids (such as lactated Ringer's solution or normal saline solution) and colloids (such as human plasma protein fraction), for volume expansion
    d. Administer blood products according to institutional protocol to replace losses and maintain HCT levels
    e. Insert a nasogastric (NG) tube for lavage with iced saline solution or water to decrease or control bleeding

CLINICAL ALERT

    f. Know that use of iced saline or water can increase the amount of bleeding
    g. Administer antacids to raise pH, thus decreasing acidity
    h. Administer antiulcer enzyme inhibitor agents, such as sucralfate, to coat the gastric mucosa
    i. Administer a histamine (H_2) receptor antagonist, such as cimetidine, ranitidine, or famotidine, to reduce gastric acid production
    j. Administer vasopressin for massive bleeding
    k. Give parenteral nutrition to meet the patient's metabolic needs
    l. Prepare the patient for pulmonary artery catheter placement to monitor fluid status and evaluate therapy
    m. Assess and document CVP, PAP, PAWP, CO, and SVR
    n. Assess and document continuous ECG rhythm; vital signs; mental status; heart, lung, and bowel sounds; urine output; and any signs and symptoms indicating changes in these parameters
    o. Measure and record all fluid losses from the GI tract
    p. Check all emesis, stool, and drainage for blood
    q. Monitor Hb and HCT results, and report abnormal values
    r. Provide comfort measures, such as oral care, and remove all soiled and odorous materials on or near the bed
    s. Provide emotional support to decrease fear and anxiety
    t. Prevent transmission of infection by washing hands thoroughly and wearing gloves if contact with blood or body fluids is likely
    u. Prepare the patient for surgical intervention for ligation of bleeding vessels, removal of the ulcer or malignant lesion, sclerotherapy (injection of a sclerosing agent that causes fibrosis) to control bleeding
    v. Teach the patient the importance of seeking medical attention if signs and symptoms of bleeding recur
    w. Teach the patient the importance of avoiding alcohol if it is a causative factor

♦ V. Acute pancreatitis

A. General information

1. Pancreatitis is an inflammatory disease of the pancreas caused by an autodigestive process of pancreatic tissue by its own enzymes
2. Trypsinogen, phospholipase, and elastase are the enzymes responsible for initiating autodigestion
3. The pancreas functions normally before and after an acute episode
4. Necrosis and hemorrhage are precursors of complete pancreatic dysfunction
5. Mortality from pancreatitis may be greater than 70% in patients with necrosis and hemorrhage
6. Respiratory failure is a common complication because the pancreas releases phospholipase, which destroys surfactant
7. Other potential life-threatening complications include intravascular coagulopathies, renal failure, circulatory collapse, and sepsis

B. Causes

1. Excessive alcohol intake (causes more than 60% of cases; more common in men)
2. Hyperlipidemia
3. Certain drugs (corticosteroids, thiazide diuretics, and estrogens)
4. Biliary tract dysfunction with reflux or stones (more common in women)
5. Viral or bacterial infection
6. Trauma
7. Surgical procedures involving the gastric, biliary, and cardiac organs

C. Assessment findings

1. Severe midepigastric or abdominal pain, often radiating to the back
2. Nausea, vomiting, and severe weight loss
3. Diarrhea
4. Fever
5. Abdominal rigidity
6. Hyperactive bowel sounds
7. JAUNDICE; discolored urine
8. Hypotension
9. Hypoventilation with crackles
10. Positive Chvostek's and Trousseau's signs if hypocalcemia is present
11. Turner's sign (bluish discoloration of lower abdomen and flanks) or Cullen's sign (discoloration in periumbilical area)

D. Diagnostic test findings

1. Serum amylase levels: elevated
2. Urine amylase levels: elevated
3. Serum glucose levels: elevated

4. Serum calcium levels: decreased
5. White blood cell (WBC) count: elevated indicates inflammation
6. Coagulation studies: decrease in platelets and fibrin
7. Hb and HCT levels: decreased if bleeding
8. Abdominal X-ray: calcification in epigastric area if process is chronic
9. ABG measurements: hypoxemia and respiratory alkalosis initially, then acidosis as the patient's condition deteriorates
10. ECG: ST-segment and T-wave abnormalities from hypoxia and widening ST segment from hypocalcemia

E. Patient care management
1. Goals
    a. Relieve pain
    b. Rest the pancreas by minimizing demands for insulin and enzymes
    c. Maintain adequate circulating fluid volume
2. Strategies
    a. Administer oxygen therapy if hypoxia is present; monitor SaO_2 with pulse oximeter
    b. Intubate and mechanically ventilate if the patient cannot maintain breathing
    c. Administer meperidine hydrochloride for pain rather than morphine, which can cause spasms of pancreatic and biliary ducts
    d. Administer I.V. fluids for hydration, volume expansion, and electrolyte replacement
    e. Administer insulin if hyperglycemia is present
    f. Insert an NG tube to relieve gastric distention and suppress pancreatic secretion
    g. Prepare the patient for pulmonary artery catheter placement to monitor fluid status and evaluate therapy
    h. Assess and document CVP, PAP, PAWP, CO, and SVR, as ordered
    i. Assess and document continuous ECG rhythm; vital signs; mental status; heart, lung, and bowel sounds; urine output; and any signs and symptoms indicating changes in these parameters
    j. Provide parenteral nutrition to support metabolic needs and defend against infection
    k. Administer antibiotics appropriate for the causative organism
    l. Limit activity to decrease metabolic demands
    m. Monitor for seizure activity
    n. Measure and record all fluid losses from the GI tract
    o. Monitor serum glucose and amylase levels, and report abnormal values
    p. Offer frequent mouth care and comfort measures when fluids are restricted or an NG tube is in place
    q. Prevent transmission of infection by washing hands thoroughly and wearing gloves if contact with blood or body fluids is likely

r. Provide emotional support to decrease fear and anxiety
s. Teach the patient the importance of avoiding alcohol if it is a causative factor

♦ VI. Hepatitis

A. General information
1. Hepatitis involves inflammation of and injury to the liver, resulting in necrosis and scarring
2. It is an infectious process that is viral in nature
3. There are five isolated types of hepatitis: A, B, C, D, and E
4. Hepatitis A virus results in the disease previously called infectious hepatitis
   a. It usually affects children and young adults
   b. It may be asymptomatic or have a rapid onset of symptoms
   c. It is transmitted by the fecal-oral route
   d. Incubation time is usually 2 to 6 weeks
   e. Infection with the hepatitis A virus is acute and appears to induce lifelong protection against subsequent infection
5. Hepatitis B virus results in the disease previously called serum hepatitis
   a. It affects all age-groups
   b. It may be asymptomatic or have a prolonged onset of symptoms
   c. It is transmitted by exchange of blood and body fluids (especially contaminated needles)
   d. Incubation time is usually 6 to 26 weeks
   e. Most adults acutely infected with hepatitis B virus recover and produce immunity from future infection; young children and few adults develop chronic infection and may die prematurely from cirrhosis or liver cancer
   f. A vaccine is available to prevent the spread of infection
6. Hepatitis C virus is associated with the majority of hepatitis cases acquired through blood transfusion; the virus also can be sexually transmitted
   a. It affects all age-groups
   b. Incubation time is usually 6 to 7 weeks but can be up to 26 weeks
   c. Patients usually develop chronic infection and are at increased risk for developing cirrhosis and liver cancer
   d. No protective antibody response has been identified after infection with hepatitis C virus
7. Hepatitis D virus is found only in those infected with hepatitis B; the hepatitis D virus requires hepatitis B virus to replicate
   a. It is transmitted by exchange of blood and body fluids
   b. Infection with hepatitis D virus can be avoided with prophylaxis against hepatitis B virus

8. Hepatitis E virus is enterically transmitted
   a. It occurs in those resistant to hepatitis A
   b. It is more common in young adults and pregnant women
   c. Incubation period is usually 2 to 8 weeks
   d. No evidence of chronic infection has been detected in long-term follow-up of patients with hepatitis E

B. Causes
1. Viral infections
2. Alcohol
3. I.V. drug use
4. Contaminated needles, water, or food
5. Blood transfusions
6. Shellfish

C. Assessment findings
1. Jaundice
2. Fatigue
3. Nausea and vomiting
4. Anorexia
5. Abdominal tenderness over liver area
6. Diarrhea with clay-colored stools
7. Dark urine
8. Headache
9. Low-grade fever

D. Diagnostic test findings
1. Serum bilirubin levels: elevated because of failure in hepatocyte metabolism
2. Serum alkaline phosphatase levels: elevated because of inability to excrete
3. Liver enzyme levels (serum aspartate aminotransferase, serum alanine aminotransferase, and lactate dehydrogenase): elevated because of inability to excrete (may be 10 times the normal values)
4. Serum antigen or antibody tests: positive for hepatitis B virus
5. Stool and serology: positive for hepatitis A virus
6. Ultrasonography: shows enlarged liver
7. Liver biopsy: confirms extent of cellular damage

E. Patient care management
1. Goals
   a. Correct the causative factors
   b. Prevent further damage and complications
2. Strategies
   a. Administer oxygen if hypoxia is present; monitor SaO_2 with pulse oximeter

TEACHING TIPS
Patient with hepatitis

Be sure to include the following topics in your teaching plan for the patient with hepatitis.

- Modes of transmission
- Methods to prevent transmission to others
- Risk of continued use of alcohol (increases morbidity and mortality)
- Community resources for alcohol and drug withdrawal programs
- Signs and symptoms of progressive hepatic disease (dark urine, ascites, fatty stools, confusion, jaundice)
- Importance of medical follow-up appointments

b. Administer I.V. fluids for hydration, volume expansion, and electrolyte replacement
c. Administer thiamine replacement if the patient is an alcoholic or if thiamine levels are deficient
d. Assess and document continuous ECG rhythm; vital signs; mental status; heart, lung, and bowel sounds; urine output; and signs and symptoms indicating changes in these parameters
e. Administer antacids and antiemetics to decrease nausea and gastric acidity
f. Administer high-calorie, high-carbohydrate diet
g. Monitor serum albumin, alkaline phosphatase, BUN, bilirubin, and other laboratory results, and report abnormal values
h. Schedule clusters of activities between rest periods to conserve the patient's energy
i. Institute protective measures to prevent skin damage, including lotion, pressure-relief devices, and position changes
j. Prevent transmission of infection by washing hands thoroughly and wearing gloves if contact with blood or body fluids is likely
k. Prepare the patient for possible liver biopsy to determine the extent of hepatic involvement
l. Provide emotional support to decrease fear and anxiety
m. Provide the patient with educational information about the importance of informing others of infection if it will have a major health effect (for teaching tips, see *Patient with hepatitis*)
n. Teach the patient the importance of avoiding alcohol and I.V. drug use if they are causative factors

CLINICAL ALERT

o. Be aware that after accidental exposure, passive immunoprophylaxis can be achieved by administration of hepatitis B immune globulin (H-BIG); this postexposure inoculation is recommended for high-risk patients

♦ VII. Hepatic failure

A. General information
1. Hepatic (liver) failure is loss of normal liver functions because of damage to and destruction of hepatocytes
2. Liver functions are complex chemical processes that include vascular control, secretory function, metabolic regulation, and storage of reserve nutrients
3. In hepatic failure, hepatocytes are progressively destroyed and replaced with fibrotic tissue
4. Approximately 75% of liver tissue can be destroyed without the patient's having experienced signs and symptoms
5. Hepatocytes can regenerate and potentially reverse cellular damage if the patient survives the acute attack

B. Causes
1. Alcoholic or Laënnec's cirrhosis
2. Hepatitis
3. GI bleeding
4. Obstructive biliary disease
5. Hypovolemia from shock or rapid diuresis
6. Infection
7. Hepatotoxic drugs, such as halothane, isoniazid, and acetaminophen
8. Poisons, toxins, drug overdose
9. Stress

C. Assessment findings
1. Jaundice
2. Anorexia or weight loss
3. Altered level of consciousness (LOC) progressing to coma
4. ASTERIXIS
5. Ascites or edema
6. Dyspnea or decreased breath sounds
7. Ecchymosis, purpura, and bleeding from the oral mucosa
8. Fever
9. Hypertension
10. Increased CO associated with decreased SVR progressing to shock
11. Fetor hepaticus (fecal odor to breath)
12. Rectal and esophageal varices
13. Endocrine changes, such as testicular atrophy and gynecomastia in males and erratic menses in females

D. Diagnostic test findings
1. Serum ammonia levels: elevated because of inability to convert to urea

2. Serum alkaline phosphatase levels: elevated because of inability to excrete
3. BUN levels: increased because of renal failure or bleeding
4. Serum bilirubin levels: elevated because of failure in hepatocyte metabolism; may indicate poor prognosis
5. Serum albumin levels: decreased and may indicate poor prognosis
6. CBC: decreased Hb and HCT levels and red blood cell (RBC) count; may reflect bleeding
7. PT: prolonged because of decrease in synthesis of vitamin K clotting factors
8. WBC count: elevated with infection
9. Hepatitis B surface antigen screen: detects active hepatitis B
10. Liver biopsy: may determine cause of dysfunction

E. Patient care management
   1. Goals
      a. Correct causative factors
      b. Prevent further damage and complications
   2. Strategies
      a. Administer oxygen to correct hypoxia; monitor SaO_2 with pulse oximeter
      b. Administer I.V. fluids for hydration, volume expansion, and electrolyte replacement
      c. Administer packed RBCs if needed for decreased HCT levels
      d. Administer fresh frozen plasma if needed for clotting factors
      e. Prepare the patient for pulmonary artery catheter placement to monitor fluid status and evaluate therapy
      f. Assess and document CVP, PAP, PAWP, CO, and SVR, as ordered
      g. Assess and document continuous ECG rhythm; vital signs; mental status; heart, lung, and bowel sounds; urine output; and any signs and symptoms indicating changes in these parameters
      h. Insert an NG tube to relieve gastric distention and to administer medications
      i. Administer thiamine replacement if the patient is an alcoholic or if thiamine levels are deficient
      j. Administer H_2 receptor antagonist to prevent gastric erosion from stress
      k. Administer neomycin to reduce ammonia-producing bacteria in the bowel
      l. Administer lactulose to induce osmotic diarrhea
      m. Administer parenteral nutrition, including a high-calorie, low-protein, low-sodium diet, if the GI tract is nonfunctional
      n. Monitor serum albumin, alkaline phosphatase, BUN, and bilirubin levels, and report abnormal values

o. Offer frequent mouth care and comfort measures when fluids are restricted
p. Institute protective measures to prevent skin damage, including lotion, pressure-relief devices, and position changes
q. Provide safety measures to prevent accidental injury from altered LOC, seizures, or coma
r. Prevent transmission of infection by washing hands thoroughly and wearing gloves if contact with blood or body fluids is likely
s. Prepare the patient for paracentesis, ultrafiltration, or peritoneal venous shunt to remove ascites
t. Prepare the patient for surgical intervention, including hepatic resection or liver transplantation
u. Provide emotional support to decrease fear and anxiety
v. Teach the patient the importance of avoiding alcohol if it is a causative factor

Points to remember

- Most acute GI bleeding is from an arterial source.
- All emesis, stool, and drainage of patients with acute GI bleeding should be checked for blood.
- GI pain in acute pancreatitis should be treated with meperidine rather than morphine, which can cause spasms of the pancreatic and biliary ducts.
- Transmission of infection can be prevented by washing hands thoroughly and wearing gloves when contact with blood or body fluids is likely.

Study questions

To evaluate your understanding of this chapter, answer the following questions in the space provided; then compare your responses with the correct answers in Appendix B, pages 286 and 287.

1. Which area of the esophagus is most often the site of esophageal varices?

____

____

2. Why is vasopressin a drug of choice for bleeding esophageal varices?______

____

____

3. Why is it necessary to use traction or tension when deflating the balloon tamponade device? ______________________________

____

____

4. What is the cause of most lower GI hemorrhages? ______________________________

____

____

5. Which enzyme initiates autodigestion of the pancreas? ______________________________

____

____

6. Why is meperidine hydrochloride the narcotic of choice for pain management in pancreatitis? ______________________________

____

____

CRITICAL THINKING AND APPLICATION EXERCISES

1. Observe an endoscopy. Describe the procedure and findings to classmates.
2. Design a pain scale and management tool for a patient with acute pancreatitis. Include the type and level of pain and the type and amount of analgesic drugs used.
3. Prepare a chart contrasting the types of hepatitis.
4. Determine what resources are available in your community to assist people undergoing alcohol or drug withdrawal.

CHAPTER 19

Female Reproductive Disorders

Learning objectives

After studying this chapter, you should be able to:

- Describe the general principles of reproductive complications.
- Identify possible causes for each type of alteration in reproductive function.
- Discuss common assessment and diagnostic test findings for the patient with a specific alteration in reproductive function.
- Describe care management for the patient with a specific alteration in reproductive function.

Chapter overview

Caring for the patient with a specific alteration in reproductive function in an emergency or critical care area requires a sound understanding of anatomy and physiology of the reproductive system. Various causes contribute to each type of alteration in reproductive function. Common assessment and diagnostic test findings are used to determine the type and extent of dysfunction. In general, care management for the patient with a specific alteration in reproductive function is aimed at early detection of deviations from normal during pregnancy and delivery. Additionally, all patient care management strategies must safeguard both the mother and the fetus while providing adequate, realistic, psychological reassurance.

I. Introduction

A. Reproductive emergencies risk the health and life of the mother and fetus

B. The emergency department nurse is likely to see the woman with reproductive risks at admission; depending on the institution, complicated pregnancies may be cared for on the obstetric floor or in the intensive care unit

C. Potential nursing diagnoses for the patient with a reproductive disorder
1. Anticipatory or dysfunctional grieving
2. Decreased cardiac output
3. Pain
4. Risk for injury

II. Anatomy and physiology

A. Structures
1. The female reproductive system includes the breasts and external and internal genital organs
2. External genital organs include the mons pubis, labia majora, labia minora, clitoris, vaginal vestibule, hymen, and Bartholin's glands
3. Internal genital organs include the vagina, uterus, fallopian tubes, and ovaries

B. Neurohormonal control
1. The hypothalamus, anterior pituitary gland, and ovaries secrete hormones that operate by positive and negative feedback mechanisms
2. The autonomic and spinal nerve pathways innervate the reproductive organs

III. Ectopic pregnancy

A. General information
1. Ectopic pregnancy involves implantation of the fertilized ovum outside the uterine cavity
2. Most ectopic pregnancies occur in the fallopian tubes, more often in the right tube than the left
3. At least 75% of ectopic pregnancies are diagnosed in the first trimester and are symptomatic

CLINICAL ALERT

4. Fetal mortality rate is close to 100%; if diagnosis is delayed, maternal morbidity rate is high

B. Causes
1. Tubal damage from pelvic inflammatory disease
2. Congenital fallopian tube abnormalities
3. Hormonal deficiencies
4. Adhesions from previous abdominal surgery

C. Assessment findings (occur only after the fallopian tube ruptures)
1. Sharp unilateral abdominal pain
2. Syncope
3. Referred shoulder pain
4. Profuse vaginal bleeding

D. Diagnostic test findings
1. Pelvic examination: pelvic mass and tenderness
2. CULDOCENTESIS: aspiration of nonclotted blood
3. Ultrasonography: ectopic location of fetus
4. LAPAROSCOPY: nonruptured tubal pregnancy, if culdocentesis is not performed
5. Laparotomy: diagnosis and opportunity for treatment
6. Complete blood count (CBC): decreased hemoglobin (Hb) and hematocrit (HCT) levels

E. Patient care management
1. Goals
   a. Control hemorrhage and replace blood loss
   b. Remove ectopic pregnancy
   c. Provide support to the patient and family
2. Strategies
   a. Type and crossmatch for possible blood transfusions to replace lost blood volume
   b. Prepare the patient and family for surgery
   c. Perform immediate laparoscopy to confirm diagnosis
   d. Consider hysterectomy for ruptured interstitial or cornual pregnancy; remove ovary if ovarian pregnancy
   e. Establish a large-bore I.V. line to gain access for adequate fluid replacement and, possibly, blood administration
   f. Assess for shock; monitor for increased heart rate, decreased blood pressure, diaphoresis, and pallor
   g. Assess and document continuous electrocardiogram (ECG) rhythm; vital signs; heart, lung, and bowel sounds; urine output; and any signs and symptoms indicating changes in these parameters
   h. Assess the patient's emotional state and coping mechanisms to evaluate the effect of losing the child

   CLINICAL ALERT

   i. Recognize that this is a crisis for the family
   j. Explain the diagnosis and implications to the patient and family to aid decision making about future pregnancies
   k. Refer the patient and family to community resources that can provide support, such as social services, counseling, and local support groups

♦ IV. Spontaneous abortion

A. General information

1. Spontaneous abortion, also called miscarriage, is an interruption of a pregnancy due to natural causes before the fetus is viable
2. It is classified as an early abortion if it occurs before the 16th week of pregnancy and as a late abortion if it occurs between 16 and 24 weeks
3. Establishing the week of pregnancy in which bleeding occurs is important in determining the woman's risk for severe bleeding
   a. Bleeding is rare before week 6
   b. Bleeding can be severest between weeks 6 and 12
   c. After week 12, although bleeding can be severe, uterine contractions help control placental bleeding
4. Spontaneous abortion is one of the most common causes of bleeding during the first trimester
5. There are six types of spontaneous abortion: threatened, imminent, complete, incomplete, missed, and recurrent

B. Causes

1. Abnormal fetal formation
2. Implantation abnormalities
3. Inadequate progesterone levels
4. Abdominal trauma
5. Maternal infection

C. Assessment findings

1. Vaginal spotting; bright red vaginal bleeding
2. Cramping, possibly progressing to uterine contractions (not present for a threatened abortion)
3. Cervical dilation (none for a threatened abortion)

D. Diagnostic test findings

1. Ultrasonography: possible implantation abnormalities
2. Pregnancy test: if pregnancy not confirmed
3. CBC: decreased Hb and HCT levels

E. Patient care management

1. Goals
   a. Identify and treat the condition promptly, and prevent hemorrhage
   b. Help the family deal with the crisis of losing a child
2. Strategies
   a. Place the woman on her side to maintain optimal placental and renal function

b. Provide fluid administration — usually with lactated Ringer's solu-tion — through a large-bore I.V. line to maintain fluid balance
c. Type and crossmatch 2 units of blood in case of hemorrhage
d. Assess for shock; monitor for increased heart rate, decreased blood pressure, diaphoresis, and pallor
e. Assess and document continuous ECG rhythm; vital signs; heart, lung, and bowel sounds; urine output; and signs and symptoms indicating changes in these parameters
f. Assess the patient's emotional state and coping mechanisms to evaluate the effect of losing the child

CLINICAL ALERT

g. Recognize that this is a crisis for the family
h. Explain the diagnosis and implications to the patient and family to aid decision making about future pregnancies
i. Refer the patient and family to community resources, such as social services, counseling, and local support groups

V. Placenta previa

A. General information
1. In placenta previa, the placenta implants in the lower uterine segment (may be total, partial, or low, according to location)
2. Because the lower uterine segment has less blood supply than the uterus, the placenta is forced to spread out over a wider area, so it approaches or covers the cervical os
3. The proximity of the placenta to the os increases the risk for infection from the vagina
4. Postpartum hemorrhage may occur with the fundus firmly contracted
5. Certain factors, such as age (35 years or older), high parity, and a history of placenta previa, may increase a pregnant patient's risk

B. Cause: unknown

C. Assessment findings
1. Painless uterine bleeding, especially in the third trimester
2. Normal uterine tone
3. LEOPOLD'S MANEUVER: the fetus is in a breech, oblique, or transverse position
4. Port wine amniotic fluid

D. Diagnostic test findings
1. Ultrasonography: location of placenta previa
2. Vaginal examination: placenta inside cervical os; because of danger of bleeding, this examination should be done only if ultrasonography is not available
3. CBC: decreased Hb and HCT levels if bleeding is present

E. Patient care management
1. Goals
   a. Identify and treat the condition promptly
   b. Prevent hemorrhage
   c. Deliver a healthy, mature neonate
2. Strategies
   a. Maintain bed rest and elevate the head of the bed
   b. Provide fluid administration — usually with lactated Ringer's solution — through a large-bore I.V. line to maintain fluid balance
   c. Type and crossmatch 2 units of blood in case of hemorrhage
   d. Consider cesarean delivery if the placenta previa is more than 30% or if excessive bleeding occurs
   e. Maintain electronic monitoring of the mother and fetus to prevent complications
   f. Assess and document continuous ECG rhythm; vital signs; neurologic status; heart, lung, and bowel sounds; urine output; fetal and maternal monitoring; and any signs and symptoms indicating changes in these parameters
   g. Weigh saturated perineal pads to assess maternal blood loss
   h. Measure fundal height to assess for rising fundus, which may reveal concealed bleeding

CLINICAL ALERT

   i. Disallow rectal or vaginal examinations to minimize the danger of bleeding

CLINICAL ALERT

   j. Prepare the patient and family emotionally and physically for delivery
   k. Recognize that this is a crisis for the family
   l. Observe for meconium in the amniotic fluid; may indicate fetal distress
   m. Provide emotional support to the patient and family

♦ VI. Abruptio placentae

A. Introduction
1. Abruptio placentae involves premature separation of the placenta from the uterine wall
2. It begins when the small arteries in the uterine wall degenerate, rupture, and hemorrhage, severely reducing blood flow to the placenta; distended by pregnancy, the uterus cannot contract and compress the torn vessels effectively, and hemorrhage continues
3. Abruptio placentae is classified as marginal, central, or complete
   a. In *marginal abruptio placentae,* bleeding between the fetal membranes and the uterine wall escapes vaginally
   b. In *central abruptio placentae,* bleeding is concealed between the uterine wall and the placenta

   c. *Complete abruptio placentae* is marked by sudden, profuse vaginal bleeding
4. Abruptio placentae may be so slight as to prevent diagnosis until after delivery or so severe as to cause serious maternal complications and fetal death

B. Causes
1. Increased intrauterine pressure from multiple pregnancy or hydramnios
2. Maternal hypertension
3. High maternal parity or age
4. Excessive maternal alcohol use or cigarette smoking
5. Abdominal trauma

C. Assessment findings
1. Dark red vaginal bleeding; quantity depends on the degree of placental separation
2. Abdominal tenderness and rigidity
3. Increased abdominal girth
4. Signs of hypovolemic shock

D. Diagnostic test findings
1. Ultrasonography: may be normal
2. Coagulation values: decreased fibrinogen and platelet levels

E. Patient care management
1. Goals
   a. Identify and treat the condition promptly
   b. Restore blood loss and prevent complications
2. Strategies
   a. Assist with fetal delivery, which may include procedures such as AMNIOTOMY, oxytocin stimulation, and cesarean delivery, depending on the patient's clinical condition
   b. Maintain electronic monitoring of the mother and fetus to detect signs of distress or abnormalities
   c. Begin fluid administration — usually lactated Ringer's solution — through a large-bore I.V. line to maintain fluid volume
   d. Type and crossmatch 3 units of blood for transfusion, if necessary
   e. Administer oxygen at a flow rate based on institutional policy and the patient's clinical condition to increase fetal oxygenation

CLINICAL ALERT

   f. Assess for early signs of disseminated intravascular coagulation, the most serious complication, such as bruising, petechiae, and bleeding from the nose, gums, or I.V. sites
   g. Assess and document continuous ECG rhythm; vital signs; neurologic status; heart, lung, and bowel sounds; urine output; fetal and maternal monitoring; and any signs and symptoms indicating changes in these parameters

h. Weigh saturated perineal pads to assess the mother's blood loss
i. Measure fundal height to detect a rising fundus, which may reveal concealed bleeding

CLINICAL ALERT

j. Assess the patient's emotional state and coping mechanisms
k. Recognize that this is a crisis for the family
l. Prepare the patient for surgery, if indicated
m. Administer medications, as ordered, for discomfort, anemia, or uterine ATONY, and document the patient's response
n. Refer the family to community resources, such as social services, counseling, and local support groups, if the fetus is nonviable

♦ VII. Pregnancy-induced hypertension (PIH)

A. Introduction

1. PIH is defined as consistent blood pressure readings of more than 140/90 mm Hg, or an increase over baseline of 30 mm Hg in systolic pressure or 15 mm Hg in diastolic pressure developing during an established pregnancy
2. PIH typically develops after 20 weeks' gestation and resolves after the 10th postpartum day
3. PIH is classified as preeclampsia or eclampsia

CLINICAL ALERT

4. A syndrome called HELLP (Hemolysis, Elevated Liver function, and Low Platelet count) has been linked with severe preeclampsia
5. PIH is a leading cause of maternal mortality
6. Risk factors associated with PIH include primigravidity, multiple fetuses, vascular disease, molar pregnancy, family history, and deficiencies in dietary protein and water-soluble vitamins

B. Cause: unknown

C. Assessment findings

1. Hypertension
2. Sudden excessive weight gain
3. Generalized edema
4. Headaches or seizures
5. Hyperreflexia
6. Blurred or double vision
7. Fetal growth retardation or fetal distress

D. Diagnostic test findings

1. Blood pressure: elevated above defined levels (definitive test)
2. Urinalysis: proteinuria
3. Serum liver function tests: elevated serum aspartate aminotransferase, serum alanine aminotransferase, bilirubin
4. Serum platelets: decreased

5. Serum creatinine level: increased
6. Serum blood urea nitrogen level: increased

E. Patient care management
1. Goals:
   a. Diagnose the condition promptly
   b. Reduce blood pressure and prevent complications
   c. Deliver a healthy, mature neonate
2. Strategies
   a. Maintain complete bed rest to minimize metabolic demands
   b. Provide electronic monitoring of the mother and fetus to detect signs of distress or abnormalities
   c. Administer a high-protein, moderate-sodium diet to prevent a dietary imbalance if the patient is alert and not having seizures
   d. Administer an anticonvulsant drug, such as magnesium sulfate ($MgSO_4$), the drug of choice

CLINICAL ALERT

      (1) Before administering $MgSO_4$, check reflexes (knee, ankle, and biceps); do not give if reflexes are absent, urine output is less than 100 ml in past 4 hours, or respirations are fewer than 12 per minute to prevent potentially life-threatening adverse reactions
      (2) Have calcium gluconate available as an antidote
   e. Administer a sedative agent, such as diazepam or phenobarbital, to encourage bed rest
   f. Administer an antihypertensive agent, such as hydralazine, to reduce blood pressure, and document the patient's response
   g. Assess and document continuous ECG rhythm; vital signs; neurologic status; heart, lung, and bowel sounds; urine output; fetal and maternal monitoring; and any signs and symptoms that indicate changes in these parameters
   h. Institute safety precautions to minimize harm to the mother and fetus: maintain seizure precautions; have emergency equipment readily available; place the patient in a darkened, quiet room, and install padded side rails
   i. If seizures occur, protect the patient and record the onset, precipitating factors, type of seizure, duration, and aftermath; reassess fetal status after every seizure
   j. Test urine for proteinuria every hour or as indicated
   k. Assess for signs of abruptio placentae (see "Abruptio placentae," pages 225 to 227)
   l. Begin preparing for delivery
   m. Discuss family planning needs with the patient and family because future pregnancy may need to be delayed

TEACHING TIPS

Managing pregnancy-induced hypertension

Be sure to include the following topics in your teaching plan during the last trimester for a patient with pregnancy-induced hypertension.

- Importance of regular blood pressure checks
- Signs and symptoms necessitating medical attention
  - Weight gain of more than 1 lb/week in the third trimester
  - Severe epigastric pain and nausea and vomiting
  - Increased shortness of breath
  - Visual disturbances, such as blurred vision or spots before the eyes
  - Severe headache
  - Decreased urine output (400 to 600 ml/day)
- Risk factors and necessary lifestyle modifications
  - Activity restriction
  - Stress management
  - Diet modification

n. Teach the patient about the need for follow-up care; ensure that the underlying cause of hypertension is unrelated to pregnancy (for tips, see *Managing pregnancy-induced hypertension*)

o. Help the patient plan an acceptable means of birth control with the understanding that the patient is not a candidate for oral contraceptives

POINTS TO REMEMBER

- Reproductive emergencies create a crisis for the mother and family and may result in fetal death.
- The patient's deep tendon reflexes should be checked before administering $MgSO_4$.
- No rectal or vaginal examinations should be performed on a patient with placenta previa.
- Disseminated intravascular coagulation is one of the most serious complications in a patient with abruptio placentae.

STUDY QUESTIONS

To evaluate your understanding of this chapter, answer the following questions in the space provided; then compare your responses with the correct answers in Appendix B, page 287.

1. Where do most ectopic pregnancies occur? ______________________

2. What assessment findings are present in placenta previa? ______________________

3. What is the pathophysiology associated with abruptio placentae? ______________________

4. What is a leading cause of maternal mortality? ______________________

5. What nursing considerations are present when $MgSO_4$ is used in the patient with PIH? ______________________

CRITICAL THINKING AND APPLICATION EXERCISES

1. Describe how a nurse would estimate blood loss in a patient with placenta previa and would determine whether that blood loss was affecting the fetus.
2. Interview a mother with PIH who has delivered a healthy infant. Ask her to describe the stress she felt because of her disorder during pregnancy.
3. Follow a patient with a reproductive emergency from admission through discharge. Develop a plan of care, including any need for follow-up and home care.

CHAPTER

20

Disorders Affecting Multiple Systems

Learning objectives

After studying this chapter, you should be able to:

- Describe the general principles of caring for a patient with a disorder affecting multiple systems.
- Identify possible causes for each type of disorder affecting multiple systems.
- Discuss common assessment and diagnostic test findings for the patient with specific disorders affecting multiple systems.
- Describe care management for the patient with a specific disorder affecting multiple systems.

Chapter overview

Disorders that affect multiple systems have a profound impact on health and organ function. Such complex, life-threatening conditions must be assessed and diagnosed rapidly and managed effectively. Critical care and emergency nurses must learn to anticipate potentially life-threatening consequences of multisystem disorders and to establish patient care priorities.

I. Introduction

A. Various conditions have a profound impact on many body systems

B. The critical care and emergency nurse must anticipate this effect by integrating information and establishing patient care priorities

C. The critical care and emergency nurse must deal with critical situations with a precision and speed not usually required in other health care settings

D. Nursing diagnoses for the patient with a disorder affecting multiple body systems relate to the systems involved

1. Decreased cardiac output (CO)
2. Alteration in tissue perfusion
3. Impaired gas exchange
4. Risk for infection
5. Fluid volume excess
6. Fluid volume deficit
7. Ineffective individual coping

II. Shock: cardiogenic

A. General information

1. Cardiogenic shock is a circulatory disturbance caused by inadequate cardiac pumping from severe left ventricular damage
2. Cardiogenic shock, as a complication of myocardial infarction (MI), typically occurs when about 40% of the left ventricular wall is impaired
3. The degree of impaired myocardial contractility is related to the size of the MI
4. Two major changes in hemodynamic performance associated with cardiogenic shock include decreased CO and increased left ventricular end-diastolic pressure
5. These changes initiate a cycle of decreased systemic perfusion, decreased coronary blood flow, increased myocardial ischemia, and reduced myocardial contractility
6. Cardiogenic shock usually is fatal if untreated; early intervention improves survival

B. Causes

1. MI
2. Chronic progressive cardiomyopathy
3. Ventricular septal rupture
4. Papillary muscle rupture
5. Ventricular aneurysm

C. Assessment findings
   1. Systolic blood pressure less than 90 mm Hg or 30 mm Hg less than baseline values
   2. Oliguria, with urine output less than 20 ml/hour (or less than 0.5 ml/kg/hour)
   3. Rapid, thready pulse
   4. Cold, clammy skin
   5. Dyspnea
   6. Tachypnea
   7. Anxiety or restlessness
   8. Confusion
   9. S_3 or S_4 heart sounds
   10. Crackles

D. Diagnostic test findings
   1. Cardiac index: less than 2.2 liters/minute/m^2
   2. Pulmonary artery wedge pressure (PAWP): greater than 18 mm Hg
   3. Chest X-ray: cardiac enlargement and signs of left ventricular failure (pulmonary congestion)
   4. Echocardiogram: abnormalities of left ventricular wall motion and valve competency
   5. Serum chemistries: increased blood urea nitrogen (BUN), creatinine, and potassium levels
   6. Urinalysis: decreased specific gravity
   7. Urine creatinine clearance: decreased
   8. Arterial blood gas (ABG) measurements: decreased pH and bicarbonate (HCO_3^-); hypoxemia

E. Patient care management
   1. Goals
      a. Improve myocardial contractility
      b. Reduce myocardial workload
      c. Decrease sodium and water retention
   2. Strategies
      a. Administer oxygen at a flow rate based on the patient's clinical condition to relieve ischemia; if gas exchange is inadequate, prepare the patient for intubation
      b. Assess and document continuous ECG rhythm; vital signs; mental status; heart, lung, and bowel sounds; urine output; and any signs and symptoms that indicate changes in these parameters
      c. Obtain ABG measurements and monitor for hypoxemia and acid-base imbalance; monitor SaO_2 with a pulse oximeter
      d. If a pulmonary artery catheter is in place, assess and document central venous pressure (CVP), pulmonary artery pressure (PAP), PAWP, CO, and systemic vascular resistance (SVR)

e. As prescribed, administer drugs to increase contractility and decrease afterload, which will improve blood pressure and CO
f. Monitor intra-aortic balloon pump, if inserted, to improve coronary artery perfusion and reduce afterload
g. Administer diuretics, as prescribed, to reduce preload and improve CO
h. Administer vasodilators, as prescribed, to reduce afterload
i. Prepare for emergency percutaneous transluminal coronary angioplasty to improve blood flow through stenotic coronary arteries
j. Recognize that emergency coronary artery bypass graft surgery may be indicated to reperfuse ischemic areas; alternatively, a left ventricular assist device or heart transplantation may be indicated

♦ III. Shock: anaphylactic

A. General information

1. Anaphylactic shock is a hypersensitivity reaction to an allergen, marked by extreme respiratory distress
2. The reaction occurs in a person who has previously been exposed to the ANTIGEN and who has built up antibodies against it
3. Anaphylactic shock is a type of distributive shock
4. Untreated, it can lead to respiratory arrest and tissue hypoxia

B. Causes

1. Drugs, most commonly penicillin
2. Anesthetic agents
3. Blood transfusions
4. Insect stings or bites
5. Foods

C. Assessment findings

1. Dyspnea
2. Air hunger
3. Complete airway obstruction
4. Systolic blood pressure less than 90 mm Hg or 30 mm Hg less than baseline value
5. Palpitations
6. Nausea and vomiting
7. Urticaria
8. Swelling of eyes, lips, tongue, hands, feet, and genitalia

D. Diagnostic test findings

1. Diagnosis is based on presenting signs and symptoms
2. Immunoglobulin E serum levels: elevated (may confirm allergic reaction as origin)

E. Patient care management
   1. Goals
      a. Maintain a patent airway
      b. Counteract the effects of anaphylaxis
   2. Strategies
      a. Prepare the patient for intubation if gas exchange is inadequate
      b. Administer epinephrine to dilate bronchioles, inhibit and counteract histamine response, and increase myocardial contractility
      c. Administer oxygen at a flow rate based on the patient's clinical condition to relieve hypoxia
      d. Assess and document continuous ECG rhythm; vital signs; mental status; heart, lung, and bowel sounds; urine output; and any signs and symptoms that indicate changes in these parameters
      e. Obtain ABG measurements and monitor for hypoxemia and acid-base imbalance; monitor SaO_2 with a pulse oximeter
      f. If a pulmonary artery catheter is in place, assess and document CVP, PAP, PAWP, CO, and SVR, as ordered
      g. Begin fluid therapy with colloids and crystalloids to restore adequate vascular volume
      h. Consider administering vasopressors if fluids are not successful
      i. Provide antihistamines to relieve itching
      j. Consider bronchodilators to relieve bronchospasm
      k. Teach the patient to identify and avoid potential causative antigens
      l. Encourage the patient to wear a medical identification bracelet and to notify medical personnel of allergy
      m. Teach the family how to use an emergency anaphylaxis kit at home and how to activate the emergency medical system

♦ IV. Shock: septic

A. General information
   1. Septic shock is a life-threatening disorder caused by a bacterium, a virus, or a fungus in the bloodstream and leading to impaired cellular functioning and altered hemodynamic status
   2. Septic shock is a type of distributive shock
   3. Septic shock is the uncontrolled progression on a continuum that begins with bacteremia and leads to septicemia and septic shock

CLINICAL ALERT

   4. A septiclike response, called systemic inflammatory response syndrome, has been seen in patients with no evidence of infection
   5. Septic shock most commonly occurs when the body's defense against infection is impaired or normal protective barriers are disrupted

6. Patients at risk include those who have recently undergone traumatic injuries, surgery, or invasive procedures and those who are malnourished, immunocompromised, or debilitated
7. Gram-negative organisms are implicated in 70% of cases (for this reason, this coverage focuses on management of gram-negative shock)
8. The urinary tract is involved in about 50% of gram-negative infections
9. Nosocomial infections are the most common cause of septic shock; broad-spectrum antibiotics may be started after cultures are obtained but before sensitivity reports are available
10. Septic shock is divided into two stages: early and late
    a. In early sepsis, beta stimulation leads to increased CO but also to decreased cardiac filling pressure and SVR because of vasodilation
    b. In late sepsis, CO decreases and filling pressure increases as the heart fails; SVR is increased because of the vasoconstriction produced by the release of catecholamines and prostaglandins

B. Causes
1. Organisms: gram-negative bacteria, gram-positive bacteria, anaerobes
2. Sources and illnesses: invasive procedures, urinary tract infection, respiratory tract infection, wounds, peritonitis, GI tract infection
3. Immunosuppressant therapy

C. Assessment findings (early phase)
1. Tachycardia
2. Systolic blood pressure less than 90 mm Hg or 30 mm Hg less than baseline
3. CO less than 4 liters/minute
4. SVR greater than 1,200 dynes/sec/cm^{-5}
5. Respiratory rate less than 12 breaths per minute
6. $PaCO_2$ greater than 45 mm Hg
7 Decreasing body temperature
8. Urine output less than 30 ml/hour
9. Decreased level of consciousness (LOC)

D. Diagnostic test findings
1. ABG measurements: respiratory alkalosis progressing to respiratory acidosis
2. Serum chemistries: increased BUN, creatinine, lactate, and potassium levels; decreased HCO_3^-
3. Complete blood count (CBC): increased leukocytes and neutrophils
4. Blood cultures: positive for causative agent
5. SVR: decreased

6. Prothrombin time (PT) and partial thromboplastin time (PTT): increased
7. Liver enzyme levels (aspartate aminotransferase, alanine aminotransferase, and lactic dehydrogenase): increased

E. Patient care management
1. Goals
a. Treat the causative organism
b. Reverse vasodilation
c. Maintain tissue perfusion
2. Strategies
a. Administer oxygen at a flow rate based on the patient's clinical condition to relieve hypoxia
b. Assess and document continuous ECG rhythm; vital signs; mental status; heart, lung, and bowel sounds; urine output; and any signs and symptoms indicating changes in these parameters
c. Obtain ABG measurements and monitor for hypoxemia and acid-base imbalance; monitor SaO_2 with a pulse oximeter
d. If a pulmonary artery catheter is in place, assess and document CVP, PAP, PAWP, CO, and SVR, as ordered
e. Administer antibiotics as prescribed to combat infection, and document the patient's response
f. If gas exchange is inadequate, prepare the patient and equipment for intubation
g. Administer fluids during the early phase; then anticipate using a potent vasoconstrictor, such as norepinephrine
h. Administer inotropic agents to augment contractility and CO
i. Consider administering steroids to decrease inflammatory response
j. Use antipyretics and cooling blankets to maintain the patient's body temperature within an acceptable range, thus decreasing metabolic demands
k. Consider nutritional support to maintain adequate nutrition if the patient's oral intake is insufficient
l. Observe for complications, including renal failure, disseminated intravascular coagulation (DIC), pulmonary atelectasis, and heart failure

CLINICAL ALERT

m. Know that experimental treatments for septic shock include naloxone, ibuprofen, and monoclonal antibodies

♦ V. Shock: hypovolemic

A. General information
1. Hypovolemic shock reduces CO and causes inadequate tissue perfusion from a loss of circulating blood volume

2. Surgical patients are at high risk because of blood loss intraoperatively and trauma from the manipulation of body tissues (see "Fluid Volume Disturbances," pages 161 to 164)

B. Causes
1. Hemorrhage
2. Burns
3. Dehydration
4. Trauma

C. Assessment findings
1. Systolic blood pressure less than 90 mm Hg or 30 mm Hg less than baseline values
2. Tachycardia
3. Decreased PAWP
4. Cool, clammy skin
5. Pallor
6. Oliguria
7. Extreme thirst
8. Irritability

D. Diagnostic test findings
1. Chest X-ray: pulmonary lesions and areas of atelectasis
2. ABG measurements: respiratory alkalosis progressing to combined respiratory and metabolic acidosis; hypoxemia
3. Serum chemistries: increased BUN, alkaline phosphatase, creatinine, lactate, and potassium levels; decreased HCO_3^- and albumin levels
4. CBC: increased hematocrit (HCT) levels

E. Patient care management
1. Goal: restore the circulating blood volume
2. Strategies
   a. Assess and document continuous ECG rhythm; vital signs; mental status; heart, lung, and bowel sounds; urine output; and any signs and symptoms indicating changes in these parameters
   b. Administer fluids (lactated Ringer's or normal saline solution) to correct fluid deficit
   c. Consider administration of colloids, as necessary
   d. Obtain ABG measurements and monitor for hypoxemia and acid-base imbalance; monitor Sa_{O_2} with a pulse oximeter
   e. If a pulmonary artery catheter is in place, assess the patient's fluid volume and document CVP, PAP, PAWP, CO, and SVR, as ordered
   f. Weigh the patient daily at the same time and on the same scale with patient wearing the same amount of clothing to evaluate fluid balance

g. Administer oxygen at a flow rate based on the patient's clinical condition to relieve ischemia
h. If gas exchange is inadequate, prepare the patient and equipment for intubation
i. In patients with trauma, surgical intervention may be necessary to find the source of bleeding

♦ VI. Shock: neurogenic

A. General information
1. Neurogenic shock causes loss of overall vasomotor tone, leading to massive vasodilation and relative hypovolemia
2. The disorder is a form of distributive shock

B. Causes
1. Deep general or spinal anesthesia
2. Brain injury to medulla
3. Spinal cord injury at T-6 or above
4. Prolonged medullary ischemia
5. Overdose of barbiturates or adrenergic and ganglionic blocking agents

C. Assessment findings
1. Warm, dry, possibly flushed skin
2. Systolic blood pressure less than 90 mm Hg or 30 mm Hg less than baseline values
3. Full, regular pulse
4. Profound bradycardia
5. Poikilothermy (body temperature that varies with environmental temperature)

D. Diagnostic test findings
1. SVR: decreased
2. ABG measurements: decreased pH and HCO_3^-

E. Patient care management
1. Goals
a. Improve vasomotor tone
b. Reverse vasodilation
c. Maintain tissue perfusion
2. Strategies
a. Assess and document continuous ECG rhythm; vital signs; mental status; heart, lung, and bowel sounds; urine output; and any signs and symptoms indicating changes in these parameters
b. Obtain ABG measurements and monitor for hypoxemia and acid-base imbalance; monitor SaO_2 with a pulse oximeter

c. If a pulmonary artery catheter is in place, assess the patient's fluid volume and document CVP, PAP, PAWP, CO, and SVR, as ordered
d. Administer oxygen at a flow rate based on the patient's clinical condition to relieve ischemia
e. Perform neurologic checks (using the Glasgow coma scale), including papillary response, and report changes from baseline
f. Administer vasopressors to reverse vasodilation
g. Administer fluids, such as crystalloids and colloids, as indicated
h. Observe for a spontaneous resolution of neurogenic shock if induced by anesthesia

♦ VII. Acquired immunodeficiency syndrome (AIDS)

A. General information

1. AIDS refers to the final stage of infection by the human immunodeficiency virus (HIV)
2. HIV is transmitted primarily through contact with infected blood, semen, and vaginal secretions as well as through breast milk
3. A retrovirus, HIV incorporates itself into normal cell ribonucleic acid, destroying normal T4 helper cells and cells with a CD4 molecule (monocytes); these cells are primarily responsible for immune surveillance and recognition of mutant (neoplastic), opportunistic, and viral organisms
4. First recognized in 1981, HIV infection results in deficiencies in cell-mediated and humoral immune responses
5. Symptoms associated with HIV infection can be categorized by cause: acute retroviral infection, neurologic disease, opportunistic infections, and specific cancers
6. High-risk groups include male homosexuals and bisexuals, I.V. drug users, hemophiliacs, people who received blood transfusions before 1985, and the sexual partners of members of these groups
7. Health care professionals have a small risk of exposure from blood-to-blood contact
8. Most commonly, HIV is diagnosed in people age 30 to 40 years
9. Once positive for HIV antibodies, about 35% of people exhibit more severe illness within 5 to 6 years and the full clinical spectrum within 8 to 9 years
10. Most AIDS patients die of opportunistic or disseminated infections

B. Causes: exposure to blood or body fluids from people who are HIV positive

C. Assessment findings
1. Fever
2. Night sweats
3. Lymphadenopathy
4. Weight loss
5. Diarrhea

D. Diagnostic test findings
1. HIV seropositive by enzyme-linked immunoadsorbent assay and Western blot test
2. Presence of antibody to HIV, which usually develops 6 to 12 weeks after exposure
3. HIV culture with presence of lymphocyte clumping
4. Polymerase chain reaction with viral deoxyribonucleic acid particles noted

CLINICAL ALERT

a. Used by sophisticated laboratories to test for HIV when other tests are inconclusive
b. May be positive as soon as 2 weeks after exposure to HIV
5. Presence of other diseases, which indicate an underlying immunodeficiency
6. Absolute T4 helper lymphocyte count, which helps in predicting symptoms and clinical problems; below 500 cells/mm^3, immune compromise begins; below 200 cells/mm^3, opportunistic infections occur
7. p24 antigen test with p24 core protein detected
8. Skin tests: failure to respond reflects impairment of T lymphocytes

E. Patient care management
1. Goals
a. Restore and maintain immunologic function at baseline levels
b. Implement treatment with antiretroviral agents
c. Prevent or manage opportunistic infections, cancer, and HIV-related clinical syndromes
2. Strategies
a. Assess and document continuous ECG rhythm; vital signs; mental status; heart, lung, and bowel sounds; urine output; note alterations in signs and symptoms
b. Implement infection prevention precautions for the immunocompromised patient (no fresh flowers, limiting venipunctures)
c. Provide incremental care and frequent rest periods to reduce fatigue and oxygen consumption in patients with anemia
d. Monitor hematologic blood tests routinely
e. Monitor patient for common opportunistic infections, such as cytomegalovirus, *Pneumocystis carinii* pneumonia, and *Candida* esophagitis

f. Encourage balanced nutrition with extra protein to enhance body repair
g. Use noninvasive monitoring devices to assess vital signs; this will help reduce disruption to rest
h. Develop a progressive activity and exercise regimen
i. Encourage family participation in care
j. Provide the patient with information about health status and support services and organizations (see Chapter 2 for information on psychosocial care)
k. Institute measures to protect health care workers
   (1) Prevent transmission of HIV in the clinical setting
   (2) Minimize patient exposure to exogenous organisms
l. Explain to the patient the rationales for protective infection-control measures
m. Follow Centers for Disease Control and Prevention (CDC) recommendations for preventing HIV transmission in health care settings
n. Follow standard precautions
   (1) Consider all body secretions, especially blood, as infectious
   (2) Wash hands before and after patient contact
   (3) Wear gloves when contact with blood or body fluids is anticipated
   (4) Wear gowns, goggles, and masks to protect against splatter during suctioning or other invasive procedures
o. Don't allow the need for infection-control precautions to interfere with establishing a therapeutic nurse-patient relationship

♦ VIII. Disseminated intravascular coagulation

A. General information
1. DIC disrupts normal coagulation, producing simultaneous clotting and bleeding
2. DIC occurs as a secondary complication of another disease process
3. Activation of the extrinsic or intrinsic coagulation pathway by the primary disease causes an abnormal acceleration of clotting
4. FIBRINOLYSIS results from the conversion of plasminogen to plasmin, a proteolytic enzyme
5. Plasmin digests fibrinogen and fibrin and produces fibrin degradation products (FDPs) or fibrin split products (FSPs)
6. FDPs have an anticoagulant effect

7. Three processes — coagulation, anticoagulation, and fibrinolysis — deplete clotting factors and predispose the patient to hemorrhage
8. Most patients with DIC have had an episode of hypotension

B. Causes

1. Trauma
2. Burns
3. Surgery
4. Anaphylactic reactions
5. Transfusion reactions
6. Shock
7. Fat or pulmonary embolism
8. Prolonged extracorporeal circulation
9. Transplant rejection
10. Cirrhosis
11. Sepsis
12. Leukemia or other cancer
13. Obstetric emergencies, such as abruptio placentae, amniotic fluid embolism, and unaborted dead fetus

C. Assessment findings

1. Sudden onset of bleeding from trauma or surgical wounds
2. Oozing from body orifices, mucosal surfaces, and venipuncture sites
3. Hematuria
4. Hematemesis
5. Hemoptysis
6. Guaiac-positive stool or gastric drainage
7. Ecchymoses
8. Petechiae or mottled skin
9. Tachycardia, hypotension, and signs of shock
10. Hypotension
11. Irritability or confusion

D. Diagnostic test findings

1. Chest X-ray: interstitial edema associated with lung microemboli
2. ECG: ST-segment changes indicating ischemia
3. ABG measurements: acidosis
4. Fibrinogen levels: decreased (fibrinogen is consumed by clot formation)
5. FDPs or FSPs: increased (produced by clot dissolution)
6. PT and PTT: increased (caused by a depletion of coagulation factors)
7. Platelet count: decreased (caused by the removal of platelets from circulation to form clots)
8. Clotting factors V and VIII: reduced
9. Peripheral blood smear: the presence of fragmented red blood cells (RBCs) (caused by the deposit of fibrin in the small blood vessels)

E. Patient care management
   1. Goal: stop the bleeding by terminating the accelerated coagulation process
   2. Strategies
      a. Treat the underlying disease process
      b. Administer oxygen if hypoxia is present
      c. Administer continuous I.V. heparin
         (1) Heparin interferes with the clotting cascade at several sites and blocks the conversion of fibrinogen to fibrin, helping to minimize clot formation
         (2) Increases risk of hemorrhaging; may be controversial
      d. Administer blood component transfusion, using fresh frozen plasma, cryoprecipitate, packed RBCs, and platelets, to replace the clotting factors. Blood replacement should follow I.V. heparin or the accelerated coagulation process will rapidly consume the blood products
      e. Obtain ABG measurements and monitor for hypoxemia and acid-base imbalance; monitor SaO_2 with a pulse oximeter
      f. If a pulmonary artery catheter is in place, assess and document CVP, PAP, PAWP, CO, and SVR, as ordered
      g. Assess and document continuous ECG rhythm; vital signs; mental status; heart, lung, and bowel sounds; urine output; note alterations in signs and symptoms
      h. Suction as necessary, taking care not to traumatize fragile tissue and trigger bleeding
      i. Before administering other drugs, determine their compatibility or incompatibility with heparin
      j. Monitor results of coagulation studies, and report abnormal values
      k. Avoid giving I.M. injections to decrease risk of hematoma
      l. Offer the patient frequent oral care, using nontraumatizing devices
      m. Institute protective measures to prevent skin damage, such as lotion, pressure-relief devices, and position changes
      n. Provide a safe environment to prevent falls, tissue injury, and bruising
      o. Prevent transmission of infection by washing hands thoroughly and wearing gloves when contact with blood or body fluids is likely
      p. Teach the patient to recognize and report the signs and symptoms of coagulopathy if they recur or if chronic conditions such as leukemia exist

IX. Burns

A. General information

1. Burns refer to any damage to the skin or body tissue caused by thermal, electrical, chemical, or radiation injury
2. Damage interferes with normal skin functions, compromises protection against infection, causes loss of body fluids, alters control of body temperature, interferes with vitamin D activation, alters sensory and excretory functions, and diminishes body image
3. The extent and depth of injury relate to the intensity and duration of exposure to the source of injury
4. Regardless of cause, basic principles of burn care are the same
5. Skin damage from burns is commonly defined in terms of the skin layers involved, either partial thickness or full thickness
   a. *Partial-thickness burns* can be further classified as superficial (or first degree) and deep partial (or second degree)
   b. *Full-thickness* (or *third-degree) burns* destroy all skin layers and may damage nerves, muscles, bones, and blood vessels
6. The extent of burns in adults can be estimated quickly by using the Rule of Nines (see *Rule of Nines,* page 246)
7. Estimating the extent of burns in children involves using the Lund and Browder chart, which considers changes in the size of body parts with growth (see *The Lund and Browder chart,* page 247)
8. Three phases of burn care include the emergent, the acute, and the rehabilitation phases
   a. The *emergent* phase begins immediately after the injury as the body reacts with an inflammatory response and a large shift of extracellular fluid to the damaged tissues; this phase usually lasts 2 to 4 days
   b. The *acute* phase occurs as the body attempts to heal the wound and prevent infection; this phase begins at the end of the emergent phase and lasts until the injury is healed (either spontaneously or with grafting)
   c. The *rehabilitation* phase occurs as the patient attempts to return to optimal level of function
9. Education on burn prevention is vital because most burns are caused by carelessness, ignorance, or curiosity

B. Assessment findings

1. Partial thickness
   a. Superficial burn: pink or red skin, small blisters, pain eased by cooling, skin blanching on pressure
   b. Deep partial burn: large blisters; edema; wet, weeping, and shiny surface; pain and sensitivity to cold air

(Text continues on page 248.)

Rule of Nines

This method for estimating the extent of an adult patient's burns divides body surface area into percentages that, when totaled, equal approximately 100%. To use this method, mentally transfer the patient's burns to the body chart shown here, then add up the corresponding percentages for each burned body section. The total, a rough estimate of the extent of the patient's burns, enters into the formula to determine initial fluid replacement needs.

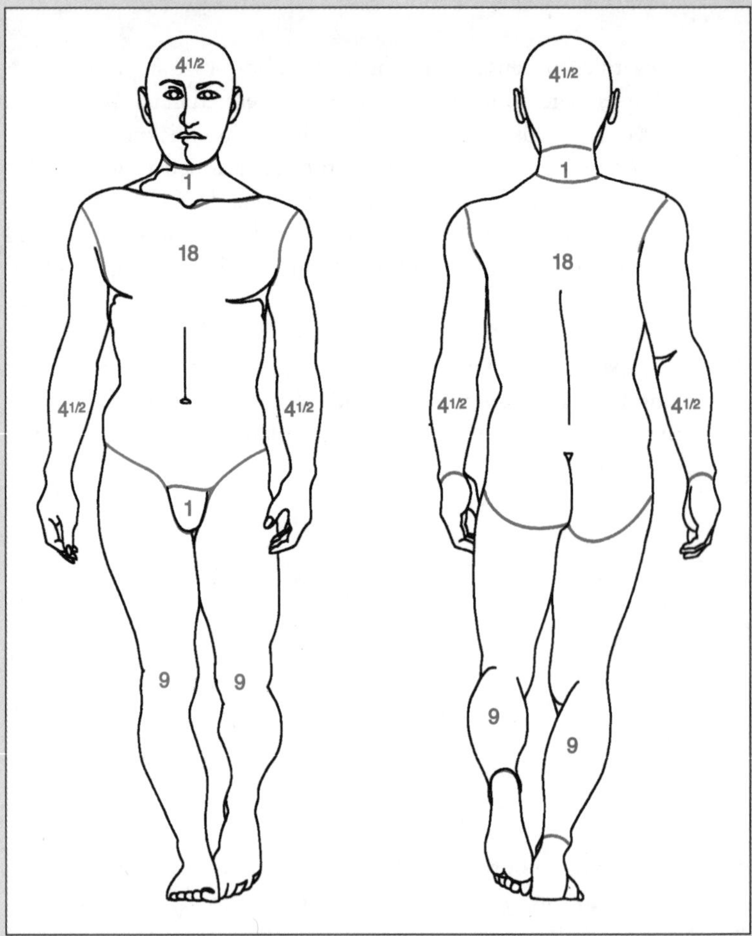

The Lund and Browder chart

The Rule of Nines is a quick way to roughly estimate the percentage of your patient's body surface that's been burned. But it can't be used for infants and children because their body section-percentages differ from those of adults. To determine the extent of an infant's or a child's burns, use the Lund and Browder chart shown here. This chart takes proportional age-size differences into account.

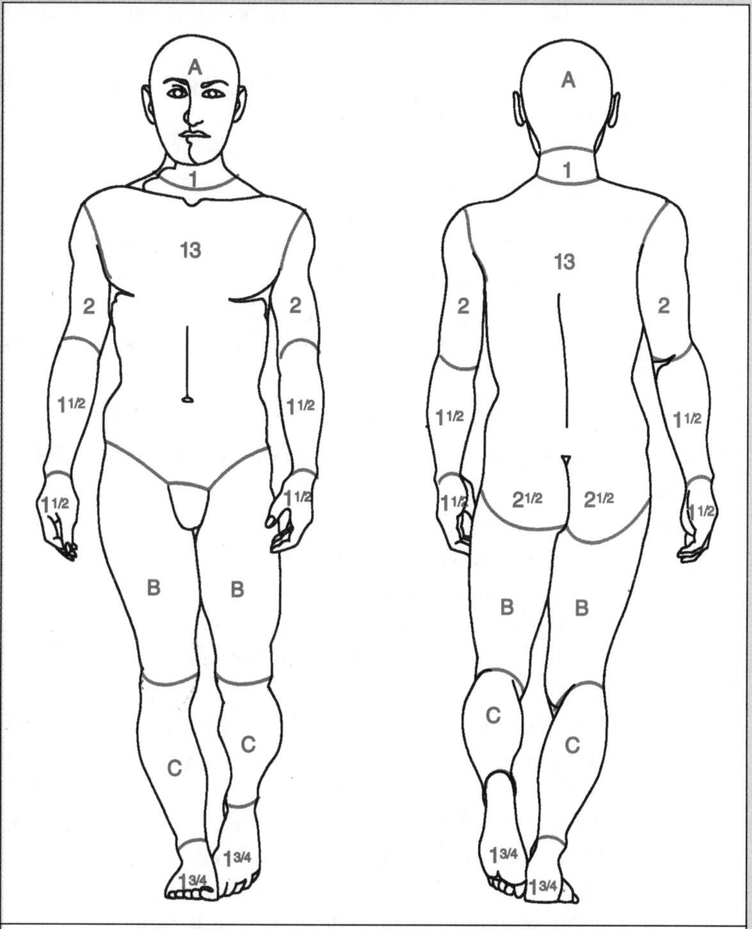

RELATIVE PERCENTAGES OF AREAS AFFECTED BY GROWTH

	At birth	1 year	5 years	10 years	15 years
A: Half of head	9½%	8½%	6½%	5½%	4½%
B: Half of thigh	2¾%	3¼%	4%	4¼%	4½%
C: Half of leg	2½%	2½%	2 ¾%	3%	3¼%

2. Full thickness
   a. Deep-red, black, or white appearance
   b. Edema
   c. Exposed subcutaneous fat layer
   d. Little or no pain
   e. Signs and symptoms of shock

C. Diagnostic test findings
1. ABG measurements: decreased partial pressure of oxygen (PaO_2) in arterial blood and increased or decreased partial pressure of carbon dioxide ($PaCO_2$) in arterial blood
2. Culture and sensitivity tests: infection (burn sepsis is defined as 10^5 microorganisms of burn tissue)
3. Carboxyhemoglobin level: positive with smoke inhalation
4. Serum chemistries: increased potassium and decreased sodium and total protein levels
5. CBC: increased HCT level initially; decreased hemoglobin (Hb)
6. Creatine kinase levels: elevated with electrical burns, with degree of elevation indicating amount of muscle injury
7. Clotting studies: decreased fibrinogen and increased FSPs detecting DIC
8. Urine studies: presence of myoglobinuria and hemoglobinuria

D. Patient care management (determined by the extent of injury and phase of care)
1. General goals of therapy
   a. Stabilize the burn victim during acute period
   b. Stop the burn process and begin wound care
   c. Have adequate wound closure with minimal scarring
   d. Have patient demonstrate positive coping skills
2. Strategies
   a. Assess and document continuous ECG rhythm; vital signs; mental status; heart, lung, and bowel sounds; urine output; and alterations in signs and symptoms
   b. If a pulmonary artery catheter is in place, assess and document CVP, PAP, PAWP, CO, and SVR, as ordered
   c. Maintain a patent airway by proper positioning, removal of secretions, and maintenance of artificial airway, if present

CLINICAL ALERT

   d. Observe for blistering of lips, singed nasal hairs, increased hoarseness, and soot in sputum, indicating injury to the respiratory tract
   e. Administer small, frequent I.V. doses of narcotics for pain relief; avoid I.M. injections for pain control until the patient is hemodynamically stable and adequate tissue perfusion is achieved

TEACHING TIPS
Patient with a burn injury

Be sure to include the following topics in your teaching plan for a patient recovering from a significant burn injury.
- Correct use of exercises and splints
- The need for foods high in protein and calories for wound healing
- Appropriate resources for assistance, including social services, rehabilitation centers, and financial services
- Medication regimen, including dosage, scheduling, and adverse effects
- Skin care measures
- Available support groups
- Medical follow-up

f. Estimate the percentage of body surface area involved using the Rule of Nines or the Lund and Browder chart
g. Begin fluid and electrolyte replacement based on institutional protocol and the patient's needs
h. Administer tetanus toxoid to combat anaerobic infections
i. Elevate the head of the bed and the burned patient's extremities to prevent edema
j. Assess wounds for local signs of infection, such as drainage, swelling, redness, or poor graft take
k. Keep the patient warm with blankets, heat lamps, and heat shields to maintain body temperature
l. Keep the patient on nothing-by-mouth status and provide low wall suction to nasogastric tube to relieve nausea and vomiting until bowel sounds return
m. Evaluate the patient's response to wound treatments, such as cleaning, debridement, whirlpool, antibacterial therapy, dressing changes, and skin grafting
n. Assess the patient's nutritional intake, providing high-calorie nutritional support to ensure that metabolic needs are met
o. Provide education and support; prepare the patient and family members for reconstruction and rehabilitation (for specific teaching tips, see *Patient with a burn injury*)

♦ X. Drug overdose (OD) or poisoning

A. General information
1. In OD and poisonings, the patient ingests more than the recommended amounts of one or more drugs, leading to altered neurologic, respiratory, or cardiac functioning

2. OD is usually an intentional, deliberate ingestion of one or more drugs
3. Poisoning is usually an accidental ingestion of a single drug
4. The following information should be obtained during the drug history:
   a. Type of drug
   b. Quantity consumed
   c. Time since ingestion
   d. Initial signs and symptoms
   e. Underlying disease
   f. Other drugs routinely taken
5. Fifteen percent of all critical care admissions can be attributed to OD and poisoning
6. Emergency department staff must be thoroughly knowledgeable about the treatments and complications of OD to ensure patient survival
7. Prognosis depends on the type and amount of drug ingested and the speed of medical intervention
8. Patients may minimize or exaggerate the amount of drug ingested, especially in intentional OD
9. The effects of injected substances, such as heroin and narcotics, can be reversed with an antidote (naloxone hydrochloride)
10. The effects of ingested substances can be treated with:
    a. Activated charcoal (if the drug is absorbed by charcoal)
    b. Induced emesis or gastric lavage (if the drug is not absorbed by charcoal)
    c. A cathartic to speed the charcoal through the gut
    d. A whole-bowel irrigation (if the drug is sustained-release)

CLINICAL ALERT

11. Ipecac syrup is the safest and most effective means to induce emesis
    a. Home remedies may be unsafe and ineffective
    b. Patient must have a gag reflex and LOC should not be depressed when administering the syrup, or aspiration may occur
12. All people who intentionally OD should be referred for psychiatric evaluation before discharge; be aware that the patient may repeat a suicide attempt while hospitalized

B. Causes
1. Suicidal or attention-seeking gesture
2. Accidental ingestion of drugs, primarily by children
3. Knowledge deficit regarding dosing of prescribed drug

C. Assessment findings: signs and symptoms vary with the type and amount of drug ingested; life-threatening findings include the following
1. Respiratory arrest
2. Cardiac arrhythmias or conduction disturbance

3. Seizures
4. Cardiovascular collapse
5. Coma

D. Diagnostic test findings
1. Drug toxicology screen of serum and urine: positive for presence, amount, and type of drug
2. Serum alcohol level: positive for presence and amount of alcohol
3. ABG measurements: mixed respiratory and metabolic acidosis with salicylate ingestion; metabolic acidosis with cyanide or carbon monoxide poisoning
4. Anion gap: elevated in ingestion of salicylates, methanol, carbon monoxide, ethanol, ethylene glycol, and paraldehyde
5. Computed tomographic scan: rules out other pathological conditions
6. Chest and abdominal X-rays: visualization of radiopaque tablets, such as iron, chloral hydrate, phenothiazines, or tricyclic agents
7. ECG: normal or reveals cardiac arrhythmias, especially ectopy

E. Patient care management
1. Goals
   a. Stabilize the patient
   b. Identify the drug ingested, prevent absorption, enhance excretion, and prevent formation of toxic metabolites
2 Strategies
   a. Maintain a patent airway and provide supplemental oxygen and respiratory support, as indicated
   b. Administer activated charcoal, induce vomiting (if the patient is conscious), or perform gastric lavage, as indicated, to reverse or eliminate the toxic substance; give no more than two doses of ipecac syrup
      (1) Document the patient's response
      (2) Give fluids or perform gastric lavage until the return is clear
      (3) Do not give ipecac syrup and activated charcoal together because the charcoal inactivates the ipecac
   c. Provide continuous cardiac monitoring because many drugs cause cardiac arrhythmias
   d. Evaluate the patient's LOC, using the Glasgow coma scale
   e. Provide suicide precautions and psychiatric evaluation, as necessary
   f. Consider hemodialysis or peritoneal dialysis if toxic substance levels require immediate elimination
   g. Administer anticonvulsants, as indicated, to minimize or prevent seizure activity

h. If restraints are necessary, place the patient in the side-lying position to prevent aspiration
i. Tailor psychosocial interventions to the patient's needs
   (1) Teach measures to prevent accidental poisoning
   (2) Refer the patient to counseling to prevent intentional OD
   (3) Provide accurate drug dose information to ensure that the patient is taking necessary medications correctly
j. Refer the patient and family members to community resources for support
k. Be sure the patient and family members know the telephone number of the nearest poison control center or crisis hot line

POINTS TO REMEMBER

- In DIC, three processes — coagulation, anticoagulation, and fibrinolysis — deplete clotting factors and cause hemorrhage.
- In all types of shock, the primary hemodynamic mechanism is inadequate oxygen delivery to the tissues.
- Anaphylactic reactions occur in people with previous exposure to an antigen who develop antibodies to the antigen.
- Nosocomial infections are the most common cause of septic shock.
- Following specific CDC guidelines and procedures for infection control is essential when caring for a patient with AIDS.
- Most burn injuries are caused by carelessness, ignorance, or curiosity; education about prevention is vital.
- All patients who intentionally OD should be referred for psychiatric evaluation before discharge.

STUDY QUESTIONS

To evaluate your understanding of this chapter, answer the following questions in the space provided; then compare your responses with the correct answers in Appendix B, page 287.

1. Which findings are characteristic of a patient with early septic shock? ______

____

____

2. Which three processes predispose the patient with DIC to hemorrhage?

____

____

3. What are the names of the coagulation pathways activated in DIC? ______

____

____

4. Which virus is responsible for causing AIDS? ______________

____

____

5. How does HIV attack and destroy cells? ______________

____

____

6. How is the extent of burn injury measured using the Rule of Nines? _____

____

____

CRITICAL THINKING AND APPLICATION EXERCISES

1. Develop a chart that shows the differences among the various types of shock with regard to cause, pathophysiology, and patient care management.
2. Imagine that you are caring for a patient with anterior chest burns that extend to the anterior surfaces of both lower extremities and the groin. Calculate the extent of burn injury using the Rule of Nines.
3. Create a chart that shows the clotting cascade and the points where heparin and warfarin sodium (Coumadin) exert their effects.
4. Develop a chart comparing the major treatments used to prevent drug absorption and removal after an OD.
5. Monitor the care of a patient with an intentional OD from admission through discharge. Develop a plan of care, including any need for follow-up and home care.

CHAPTER 21

Trauma

Learning objectives

After studying this chapter, you should be able to:

- Describe the general principles of trauma.
- Identify possible causes for each type of trauma.
- Discuss common assessment and diagnostic test findings for the patient with a specific traumatic injury.
- Describe care management for the patient with a specific traumatic injury.

Chapter overview

Critical care and emergency nurses function as an integral part of the trauma team. Various causes contribute to each type of traumatic injury. Common assessment and diagnostic test findings are used to determine the type and extent of the injury. Regardless of the cause, trauma creates the potential for significant complications and life-threatening damage. The degree of trauma depends on the nature of the force (blunt or penetrating) and the body area affected. In general, care management for the patient with trauma centers on supporting the patient's vital functions, maintaining an adequate airway and oxygenation, correcting the injury, and minimizing the consequences of the traumatic injuries.

♦ I. Introduction

A. Definition
1. Trauma is injury from force; it may be accidental, self-inflicted, or an act of violence that affects multiple systems and requires immediate, specialized interventions to prevent loss of limb or life
2. Victims commonly have injury to more than one body system
3. It is the leading cause of death for people age 1 to 44 years
4. The emergence of trauma care centers with capabilities of sophisticated emergency interventions has greatly decreased mortality and morbidity rates from traumatic injury

B. Causes
1. Motor vehicle accidents, including auto, motorcycle, and pedestrian
2. Gunshot wounds
3. Stab wounds with knives or other sharp objects
4. Falls
5. Sports-related injuries

C. Types
1. Trauma is classified as blunt or penetrating
2. *Blunt trauma* is associated with motor vehicle accidents and falls
3. *Penetrating trauma* is associated with injuries, such as stab wounds, gunshot wounds, and impalement

D. Risk factors commonly associated with trauma
1. Alcohol and drug use
2. Sex: males have twice the risk of fatal injury as females
3. Age: people age 15 to 24 years have the highest number of traumatic injuries; elderly people have the highest number of fatal injuries

E. Assessment findings

CLINICAL ALERT

1. Assessment findings depend on the systems that are injured
2. Specific nursing priorities always should be applied
   a. Maintain optimal airway, ventilation, and oxygenation
   b. Monitor for shock
   c. Restore circulating blood volume and tissue perfusion if shock occurs
   d. Correlate the mechanism of injury with the patient's clinical presentation
   e. Remain alert for new signs of injury
   f. Restore maximum mobility
   g. Strengthen muscle groups involved in weight bearing and range of motion
   h. Prevent orthopedic complications
   i. Facilitate effective coping
   j. Prevent or minimize complications

F. Potential nursing diagnoses for the patient experiencing trauma
   1. Ineffective airway clearance
   2. Ineffective breathing pattern
   3. Impaired gas exchange
   4. Decreased cardiac output
   5. Altered tissue perfusion
   6. Fluid volume deficit
   7. Impaired physical mobility
   8. Pain
   9. Risk for infection
   10. Sensory or perceptual alterations

♦ II. Head trauma

A. General information
   1. Head trauma occurs after blunt or penetrating injuries to the cranial or cerebral structures
   2. Head trauma includes skull fractures and damage to brain tissue
   3. Types of head injuries include CONCUSSION, CONTUSION, cranial fractures, epidural or subdural hematoma, subarachnoid hemorrhage, and herniation
   4. Abnormal flexion (decorticate positioning) is seen in head-trauma patients with hemispheric dysfunction
   5. Abnormal extension (decerebrate positioning) is seen in head-trauma patients with brain stem injury

B. Causes
   1. Acceleration head injury is caused by a moving object striking the head
   2. Deceleration head injury is caused by the head striking a stationary object

C. Assessment findings
   1. Concussion
      a. Nausea
      b. Vomiting
      c. Amnesia
      d. Dizziness
      e. Irritability
      f. Sluggishness
      g. Disorientation or confusion
      h. Visual disturbances
   2. Contusion
      a. Altered level of consciousness (LOC)
      b. Nausea
      c. Vomiting

   d. Visual disturbances
   e. Weakness
   f. Ataxia
   g. Speech problems
   h. Hemiparesis
   i. Seizures
3. Cranial fractures (findings depend on type and site of fracture)
   a. Altered LOC
   b. Headache
   c. Swelling
   d. Hematoma
   e. Pain
   f. Nausea
   g. Vomiting
   h. Diaphoresis
   i. RHINORRHEA or otorrhea
   j. Periorbital ecchymosis or other evidence of bleeding
4. Epidural hematoma (rapid deterioration)
   a. Altered LOC
   b. Headache
   c. Hemiparesis
   d. Ipsilateral fixed, dilated pupil
   e. Bradycardia
   f. Hypertension
5. Subdural hematoma (similar to cardiovascular accident, tumor, or senility)
   a. Headache
   b. Fever
   c. Unilateral pupil dilation
   d. Papilledema
   e. Hemiparesis or hemiplegia
6. Subarachnoid hemorrhage
   a. Piercing headache
   b. Nuchal rigidity
   c. Photophobia
   d. Nausea
   e. Vomiting
   f. Delirium
   g. Altered LOC
   h. Syncope
   i. Irritability
   j. Coma
   k. Respiratory distress
   l. Dilated pupils

m. Papilledema
n. Retinal hemorrhage
o. Focal motor signs, such as twitching
p. Seizures

7. Herniation
   a. Altered LOC
   b. Hemiparesis
   c. Respiratory distress
   d. Positive Babinski's reflex
   e. Pupillary changes

D. Diagnostic test findings

1. X-rays: reveal spinal, cervical, or skull fracture
2. Computed tomographic (CT) scan: identifies type, location, and extent of injury
3. Cerebral angiography: locates area of injury
4. EEG: locates area of irritability; shows absence of brain activity; determines presence of brain death

E. Patient care management

1. Goals
   a. Control intracranial pressure (ICP)
   b. Prevent secondary injury and complications
2. Strategies
   a. Monitor ICP to maintain cerebral perfusion pressure at 80 to 100 mm Hg
   b. Treat increased ICP by elevating the head of bed, loosening any tight garments around the neck that might impede venous return, and checking for other causes of increased ICP, such as abdominal or bladder distention and anxiety
   c. Maintain normotensive blood pressure because both hypotension and hypertension can increase cerebral edema
   d. Administer I.V. fluids (dextrose 5% in water [D5W] with normal saline solution; plain D5W can cause cerebral edema)
   e. Maintain normal body temperature to prevent hyperthermia, which increases metabolic demand
   f. Administer anticonvuslants to prevent seizures (may be given prophylactically)
   g. Administer diuretics and glucocorticoids to decrease cerebral edema and ICP
   h. Administer atracurium besylate (Tracrium) or cisatracurium besylate (Nimbex) with sedation to decrease cerebral oxygenation demands

CLINICAL ALERT

   i. Avoid the use of narcotics because they mask changes in LOC and impair neurologic assessment

j. Monitor arterial blood gas (ABG) measurements to maintain levels of partial pressure of carbon dioxide in arterial blood between 30 and 35 mm Hg because higher levels increase ICP; monitor SaO_2 with a pulse oximeter
k. Avoid coughing exercises, which increase ICP
l. Test drainage from the nose or ears for glucose (tests positive if drainage is cerebrospinal fluid [CSF])
m. Assess neurologic status and LOC frequently to detect subtle changes
n. Prepare the patient for surgical intervention, if necessary, to evacuate hematoma, elevate depressed skull fracture, remove foreign objects, and repair tears or aneurysm
o. Encourage the patient to report any aura that precedes seizure activity
p. Encourage the patient's participation in self-care and rehabilitation

♦ III. Facial trauma

A. General information
1. Facial trauma is classified by the side of the face affected and the bones involved, such as mandibular, orbital, maxillary, zygomatic, or nasal fracture
2. Because spinal cord injuries and skull fractures often accompany facial fractures, stabilizing the head and neck is essential until cervical fracture is ruled out
3. Displacement of nasal bones or cartilage can cause airway obstruction, is a potential source of infection, and can cause cosmetic concerns

CLINICAL ALERT

4. The first priority in the management of facial trauma is assessing airway patency
5. Because the face is vascular, substantial bleeding commonly accompanies facial trauma

B. Causes
1. Motor vehicle accidents
2. Violence
3. Falls
4. Sports-related injuries

C. Assessment findings
1. Soft-tissue trauma
2. Bleeding
3. Asymmetrical facial structures
4. Pain
5. Unequal eye movement or changes in vision
6. Leakage of CSF through the nose or ear

TEACHING TIPS

Patient with intermaxillary fixation

Be sure to include the following topics in your teaching plan for a patient who has undergone an intermaxillary fixation.

- Instructions that the mouth cannot be opened with jaws wired together
- Use of relaxation techniques and nose breathing if a panic attack occurs
- Use and proper location of wire cutters
- Need to carry wire cutters with the patient at all times
- Measures to take if the patient vomits
  - Sitting upright and bending head forward
  - If unable to expel the vomitus, cutting the wires that hold the jaws together, especially if airway clearance is a problem
- Strict oral care with a soft toothbrush or tooth swabs
- Refraining from use of an oral irrigating device until permitted by the doctor
- Adequate calories through a liquid diet
- Avoidance of swimming and alcohol consumption

D. Diagnostic test findings: facial X-rays identify the location and type of fracture

E. Patient care management

1. Goals
   a. Maintain a patent airway
   b. Restore any facial deformity
   c. Restore functional ability
2. Strategies
   a. Maintain patent airway
   b. Assess and document continuous electrocardiogram (ECG) rhythm; vital signs; mental status; heart, lung, and bowel sounds; urine output; and signs and symptoms that indicate changes in these parameters
   c. Provide nutritional support
   d. Provide psychological support to the patient and family
   e. Alleviate severe pain with analgesics or narcotics
   f. Assess vision and extraocular movements in patients with orbital and maxillary fractures
   g. Observe for neurologic changes

CLINICAL ALERT

   h. Be aware that drainage from the nose or ear can be assessed for glucose using Ketostix or Testape
      (1) CSF contains glucose, whereas discharge from the nose or ear does not
      (2) CSF also dries in concentric halolike rings on bed linen

i. Prepare the patient for possible intermaxillary fixation, and provide instruction on care measures after surgery (for specific teaching tips, see *Patient with intermaxillary fixation*)

♦ IV. Spinal cord injury

A. General information

1. Spinal cord injury is trauma to the spinal cord caused by hemorrhage, concussion, contusion, laceration, or diminished blood supply
2. Spinal cord injury may be referred to by type and cause as complete or incomplete or by level of injury
3. Because of the greater range of mobility in the vertebral column in certain areas, the vertebrae most commonly injured include the 5th, 6th, and 7th cervical; the 12th thoracic; and the 1st lumbar
4. Spinal cord injury severity depends on the spinal area injured
5. The major mechanisms of spinal cord injuries include hyperextension, hyperflexion, and compression

CLINICAL ALERT

6. Prompt and proper handling of the patient at the accident scene can reduce further damage and preserve remaining neurologic function
7. Of the 15,000 to 20,000 patients who sustain spinal cord injury each year, approximately 50% are rendered quadriplegic and the other 50% are paraplegic
8. Most patients with injury at or above T-6 experience autonomic dysreflexia
   a. Autonomic dysreflexia is a life-threatening response to a stimulus by the autonomic nervous system, most commonly resulting from a stimulus to the bladder
   b. Classic signs and symptoms include headache, hypertension, cutaneous vasodilation, and diaphoresis above the injured spinal cord area
9. Although the life expectancy of a patient with a spinal cord injury is estimated to be only 5 years less than a person who has not sustained a similar injury, quality of life is a major concern

B. Causes

1. Motor vehicle accidents
2. Gunshot wounds
3. Diving accidents
4. Sports-related injuries
5. Falls

C. Assessment findings: depend on location and type of injury

1. Neck or back pain
2. Vertebral tenderness or deformity
3. Extremity numbness or tingling
4. Muscle weakness or paralysis

5. Asymmetrical reflexes or absence of reflexes
6. Bowel and bladder incontinence
7. Hypotension
8. Bradycardia
9. Respiratory insufficiency (see *Guide to motor and sensory impairment in spinal cord injury*)

D. Diagnostic test findings
1. Spinal X-ray: change in vertebral positioning and cord impingement
2. CT scan: change in vertebral positioning and cord impingement
3. Magnetic resonance imaging: cord edema, necrosis, impaired blood flow in spinal cord
4. Myelography: herniated intervertebral disks or blocked CSF flow
5. Evoked potential studies and electromyography: area of spinal cord lesion
6. Pulmonary fluoroscopy: measured degree of diaphragmatic movement in patients with high cervical injuries

E. Patient care management
1. Goals
   a. Immobilize the patient
   b. Restore normal position
   c. Stabilize the vertebral column
   d. Prevent complications
2. Strategies
   a. Stabilize the patient's spine to prevent further damage
   b. Use traction, such as Harrington and Lanque, for thoracolumbar injury immobilization
   c. Consider special devices for immobilization, such as plaster jacket, Jewett nail, and Weiss spring
   d. Aid immobilization with bed frame devices with or without traction, such as Stryker frame or kinetic beds with halo traction
   e. Anticipate surgery for spinal fracture or cord compression
   f. Maintain patent airway for adequate oxygenation
   g. Consider use of a megadose corticosteroid, such as methylprednisolone sodium succinate (Solu-Medrol), on a 24-hour protocol
   h. Consider using kinetic beds to help prevent complications of bed rest and to promote peristalsis and postural drainage
   i. Alleviate severe pain with analgesics and narcotics
   j. Control muscle spasms with the use of muscle relaxants, such as baclofen

CLINICAL ALERT

   k. Assess the patient for signs and symptoms of ascending cord edema, including decreased sensory and motor loss greater than previously documented, change in respiratory pattern, and difficulty swallowing

Guide to motor and sensory impairment in spinal cord injury

SPINAL AREA AFFECTED	TYPE OF MOTOR LOSS	AREA OF SENSORY LOSS (Pain, Temperature, Touch, and Pressure)
C-1 to C-4	Diaphragm paresis Intercostal paralysis Flaccid total paralysis in skeletal muscles below neck	Neck and below
C-5 to C-8	Intercostal paralysis Paralysis below shoulders and upper arms	Arms and hands, chest, abdomen, and legs
T-1 to T-6	Paralysis below midchest	Below midchest
T-7 to T-12	Paralysis below waist	Below waist
L-1 to L-3	Paralysis in most leg muscles and in pelvis	Lower abdomen and legs
L-4 to L-5	Paralysis in lower legs, ankles, and feet	Parts of lower legs and feet
S-1 to S-5	Ataxic paralysis of the bladder and rectum Paralysis of feet and ankles	Posterior inner thigh, lateral foot, perineum

l. Evaluate for signs of autonomic dysreflexia; place the patient in a sitting position, correct the offending stimulus, and notify the doctor

m. Minimize complications of bed rest
   (1) Turn the patient frequently
   (2) Perform active and passive range-of-motion exercises
   (3) Apply antiembolism stockings
   (4) Maintain adequate hydration
   (5) Use a pressure-relief mattress or therapeutic bed

CLINICAL ALERT

n. Do not turn the patient before the spinal cord has been stabilized

o. Support the patient's psychosocial needs related to sexuality, self-esteem, and altered body image; help the patient and family cope, accept the changes, and plan for the future

p. Begin bowel and bladder retraining program, as indicated, to achieve regularly predicted elimination and prevent bladder infection

q. Direct the patient and family to community resources, such as social services, counseling, spinal cord associations, local support groups, and visiting nurses
r. Have the patient and family demonstrate the use of assistive devices and perform exercises that promote maximum functioning
s. Involve the patient and family in decisions regarding care and referral to rehabilitation centers

♦ V. Chest trauma

A. General information
1. Chest injuries are the leading cause of death in trauma victims
2. Types of chest injuries include rib fractures (most commonly ribs 5 through 9), FLAIL CHEST, myocardial or pulmonary contusion, cardiac tamponade, open pneumothorax, and hemothorax

CLINICAL ALERT

3. Penetrating objects should be removed by the doctor only after bleeding is controlled because they can have a sealing effect and their removal can produce uncontrollable bleeding or pneumothorax

B. Causes
1. Chest trauma occurs after a blunt or penetrating injury to the chest, which may involve damage to the bony structures of the thorax, the heart, or the lungs
2. Both blunt and penetrating injuries can produce pneumothorax

C. Assessment findings
1. Shortness of breath
2. Chest pain, especially with respirations
3. Tachypnea, nasal flaring, and other signs of ventilatory distress
4. Paradoxical chest wall movement (with flail chest)
5. Paradoxical pulse and blood pressure (decreased quality of pulse and blood pressure with inspiration as a result of increased intrathoracic pressure caused by accumulation of fluid in the chest cavity)
6. Hemoptysis
7. Diminished breath sounds
8. Tracheal deviation with tension pneumothorax
9. Subcutaneous crepitations

D. Diagnostic test findings
1. Chest X-ray: fractures and air or fluid in the pleural space
2. ABG measurements: acid-base imbalances and presence of hypoxemia
3. ECG: arrhythmias; ischemic changes with trauma to the coronary arteries
4. Complete blood count (CBC): decreased hemoglobin (Hb) and hematocrit (HCT) levels

E. Patient care management
1. Goal: to prevent respiratory compromise and complications from the injury
2. Strategies
   a. Maintain patent airway
   b. Assess and document continuous ECG rhythm; vital signs; mental status; heart, lung, and bowel sounds; urine output; and any signs and symptoms that indicate changes in these parameters
   c. Replace lost blood with whole blood or packed cells
   d. Prepare the patient for chest tube insertion to remove accumulated fluid or air from the chest and allow reexpansion of the lung
   e. Obtain ABG measurements and monitor for hypoxemia and acid-base imbalance; monitor SaO_2 with a pulse oximeter
   f. If a pulmonary artery catheter is in place, assess and document central venous pressure, pulmonary artery pressure, pulmonary artery wedge pressure, pulmonary vascular resistance, and systemic vascular resistance
   g. Prepare the patient for surgical intervention to stabilize flail chest or to evacuate massive hemothorax or tamponade
   h. Manage the patient's pain with nonnarcotics or intercostal nerve block so that respiration is not depressed
   i. Maintain patency and proper functioning of chest tube drainage system to ensure evacuation of drainage and air
   j. Monitor chest tube drainage for amount and color and document
   k. Be aware that autotransfusion of chest tube drainage may be used
   l. Provide chest tube dressing care according to institutional policy to prevent infection and promote healing
   m. Teach the patient to use breathing techniques to promote lung expansion and healing

♦ VI. Abdominal trauma

A. General information
1. More than 50% of patients with blunt trauma to the abdomen also have injury to the head, chest, or extremities
2. Abdominal trauma commonly causes massive blood loss and shock
3. Injury to retroperitoneal structures, such as the pancreas and duodenum, may cause blood loss of up to 4 liters, which may not be detected immediately
4. The spleen is one of the most frequently injured organs, which may cause massive hemorrhage
5. Injury to the abdominal aorta, inferior vena cava, or hepatic vessels may cause rapid, massive bleeding

B. Causes
1. Abdominal trauma occurs after a blunt or penetrating injury to the abdomen, which may cause injury to internal organs
2. Solid organs, such as the spleen, pancreas, kidneys, and uterus, typically suffer penetrating trauma
3. Hollow organs, such as the stomach, bladder, and intestines, typically suffer blunt trauma

CLINICAL ALERT

4. Abdominal trauma may also result in pelvic fracture

C. Assessment findings

CLINICAL ALERT

1. Findings may vary considerably
2. Absence of signs and symptoms does not exclude major injury
   a. Abdominal pain, ranging from mild to severe
   b. Respiratory distress from abdominal distention
   c. Signs of hypovolemia, such as decreased blood pressure, tachycardia, and pallor
   d. Wounds
   e. Abrasions
   f. Bruising on the abdomen
   g. Absent or decreased bowel sounds
   h. Decreased LOC
   i. Abdominal rigidity

D. Diagnostic test findings
1. X-rays: fractures, free air, fluid, or foreign objects
2. CT scan: intraperitoneal and retroperitoneal bleeding
3. CBC: decreased Hb and HCT levels
4. White blood cell count: increased, indicating infection
5. Serum glucose levels: elevated because of catecholamine release
6. Serum amylase levels: elevated with injury to the pancreas and small bowel
7. Liver enzymes levels (serum aspartate aminotransferase, serum alanine aminotransferase, and lactate dehydrogenase): elevated, reflecting hepatic injury from trauma or ischemia
8. Peritoneal lavage: intra-abdominal bleeding

E. Patient care management
1. Goals
   a. Correct volume deficit
   b. Prevent complications of shock and infection
2. Strategies
   a. Administer immediate fluid resuscitation with warmed saline or lactated Ringer's solution (may require use of pressure bags or infusion pumps to speed replacement)
   b. Replace lost blood with fresh whole blood; autotransfusion is avoided because of the risk of contamination

c. Apply pneumatic antishock garment to stabilize fractures
d. Evaluate wound for signs of evisceration; if present, cover with a sterile, wet saline dressing and do not attempt to replace the eviscerated tissue
e. Insert a nasogastric tube to decompress the stomach and remove gastric contents
f. Insert a urinary catheter to monitor renal function and aid in assessing genitourinary injury
g. Administer empiric antibiotics prophylactically because of high probability of infection
h. Administer nonnarcotic analgesics for pain management because narcotics decrease respiratory effort and alter sensorium
i. Administer parenteral nutrition if GI function is impaired; initiate promptly to meet the patient's metabolic needs
j. Prepare the patient for surgical intervention as indicated for wounds invading the peritoneum, GI hemorrhage, free air in abdomen, evisceration, massive hematuria, or positive diagnostic peritoneal lavage
k. Teach the patient to identify the signs and symptoms of possible bowel obstruction or infection that require medical attention

♦ VII. Limb trauma

A. General information
1. Limb trauma occurs in all age-groups and is a major source of disability
2. Most common types of limb trauma are strains, sprains, and fractures
3. Surface trauma is commonly seen with limb trauma
4. Limb trauma can result in an open wound that undergoes repair
5. Types of wound repair include the following
   a. Primary intention: margins of the wound are closely opposed and have limited cell death and minimal loss of tissue
   b. Secondary intention: margins of the wound are unopposed, with the defect containing more bacteria, debris, and exudate than wounds closed by primary union
   c. Tertiary intention: surgical closure of the wound after delaying primary wound closure; the wound is left open until infection is absent, edema has subsided, and debris has been removed
6. Wound infection and thorough cleaning of the wound site are essential to prevent infection
7. Soap solutions, such as Betadine, pHisoHex, and Hibiclens, can be toxic to cells and impair local defenses and wound healing

B. Causes
1. Limb trauma occurs after a blunt or penetrating injury to the upper or lower extremities
   a. Strains are stretch injuries that occur to the muscle at the tendon site
   b. Sprains are ligament injuries that occur from a force greater than that which causes a strain
   c. Strains and sprains are caused by any kind of movement or wrenching force
   d. Fractures are a disruption or break in a bone; they commonly are caused by a force or penetrating object that is sufficient to crack or break the bone
2. Prompt management is essential to prevent additional damage or loss of the limb
3. Surface trauma may result from abrasions, lacerations, puncture injuries, crushing wounds, or human or animal bites

C. Assessment findings
1. Strains and sprains
   a. Pain
   b. Swelling
   c. Point tenderness
   d. Discoloration
   e. Muscle spasm
   f. Brief loss of function
2. Fractures
   a. Pain
   b. Swelling
   c. Tenderness
   d. Discoloration
   e. Muscle spasm
   f. Loss of movement
   g. Deformity or angulation of limb
   h. Protrusion of bone fragments (compound fracture)

D. Diagnostic test findings: limb X-ray identifies the location and type of fracture (no specific tests for strains or sprains)

E. Patient care management
1. Goal: immobilize the affected area to allow healing and prevent further injury
2. Strategies
   a. Immobilize the strain or sprain with a compression bandage
   b. Immobilize the limb above and below the fracture site, using a splint, cast, surgical pins, sling, or traction

c. Apply a cold pack intermittently for 24 to 48 hours to decrease swelling
d. Assess limb color, temperature, capillary refill, pulses below the injury, and sensation to determine neurovascular status
e. Elevate the limb to promote venous return and decrease edema
f. Administer analgesics for pain relief
g. Anticipate administering tetanus toxoid injection if more than 5 years have elapsed since patient's last dose
h. Prepare the patient for surgery if an open reduction is necessary to stabilize the fracture
i. Provide alternate means of mobility, such as crutches or a wheelchair
j. Instruct the patient to avoid weight bearing for 24 to 48 hours after experiencing a strain or sprain
k. Teach the patient the importance of following instructions for activity limitation or exercise to restore limb function

♦ VIII. Rape trauma

A. General information

1. Rape is unlawful sexual intercourse without consent
2. Rape is a legal term, not a medical diagnosis, and its definition may vary from state to state
3. The involved parties may be men or women of any age
4. The victim is usually female
5. Rape itself is rarely a medical emergency unless rape-related trauma, such as stab wounds, lacerations, and fractures, exists

CLINICAL ALERT

6. Rape trauma represents a personal emergency for the victim and family
7. Incidence is difficult to determine because many rapes go unreported

B. Causes

1. Deviant behavior

CLINICAL ALERT

2. Alcohol use (often precedes rape)
3. Motivation generally related to expression of anger or power, not sexual satisfaction

C. Assessment findings

1. Severe emotional reaction
2. Vaginal or rectal bleeding
3. Vaginal, abdominal, or rectal pain
4. Tachycardia
5. Diaphoresis
6. Semen and blood stains on the victim's clothing
7. Bruises, cuts, or other injuries

D. Diagnostic test findings
1. Constitute legal evidence
2. Aspirated or scraped specimens from involved orifices: the male assailant's motile sperm and blood group antigen and the presence of acid phosphatase in the semen
3. Pubic hair scrapings: presence of the assailant's pubic hair
4. Fingernail scrapings: presence of the assailant's skin and blood type

E. Patient care management
1. Goals
   a. Provide emergency intervention with emotional support
   b. Collect objective evidence if the victim wants to prosecute
   c. Administer prophylactic treatment for tetanus (if open wounds are present), infection, venereal disease, and pregnancy
2. Strategies
   a. Keep in mind that the victim's informed consent is necessary for examination and treatment as well as for the collection and release of evidence to authorities
   b. Follow state law for collection of evidence and hospital protocol for the care of a rape victim
   c. Notify police, but recognize that the victim cannot be forced to talk to them
   d. Provide a person to remain with the victim at all times in a quiet, private, and nonthreatening environment
   e. Perform a thorough examination of the victim, and treat any secondary complications
   f. Record a history of the incident as well as a sexual history, including birth control measures, date of last menstrual period, and pertinent medical history
   g. Make sure all specimen containers are properly labeled, include the initials of someone present during the examination, and are sealed with lids
   h. Arrange for immediate patient counseling; put the patient in contact with a rape hot line counselor or rape crisis center
   i. Consider use of antibiotics if circumstances warrant (for example, if the rape victim suffered a human bite)
   j. Provide protection against sexually transmitted diseases by administering penicillin and probenecid
   k. Administer drugs, such as diethylstilbestrol, to protect against pregnancy if the female victim is not using reliable contraception
   l. Ensure that the victim has a family member or friend to stay with after hospital discharge

m. Provide all instructions and appointment information in writing so the victim will remember after the emotional crisis of rape
n. Make sure the victim understands the importance of medical follow-up to reevaluate the possibility of venereal disease and pregnancy

POINTS TO REMEMBER

- Victims of trauma commonly have injury to more than one body system.
- Narcotics prevent detection of changes in LOC and impair neurologic assessment.
- Any chest injury is critical because chest injury is the leading cause of death for trauma victims.
- Abdominal trauma may produce massive bleeding that is difficult to detect.
- Examination and treatment of a rape victim as well as collection of evidence and its release to authorities require the victim's informed written consent.

STUDY QUESTIONS

To evaluate your understanding of this chapter, answer the following questions in the space provided; then compare your responses with the correct answers in Appendix B, page 288.

1. What is the difference between an acceleration and a deceleration head injury? ____________________

____

____

2. Which type of posturing is seen in patients with an injury to the brain stem?

____

____

3. Which assessment findings are common to all types of head injuries? ______

____

____

4. Which position facilitates cerebral venous return and assists in the control of ICP? ____

____

____

5. Why are nonnarcotic analgesics used for pain management in patients with chest and abdominal trauma? ____

____

____

6. What is the immediate nursing action for wound evisceration? ___________

____

____

7. What is the immediate patient care management goal for limb trauma? ___

____

____

8. Which diagnostic tests provide legal evidence in rape trauma cases? ______

____

____

CRITICAL THINKING AND APPLICATION EXERCISES

1. Develop a chart outlining patient care management strategies for a patient with a C-3 spinal cord injury.
2. Follow a patient with a chest trauma from admission through discharge. Develop a plan of care, including any need for follow-up and home care.
3. Interview a rape crisis counselor about the key concerns of rape victims.
4. List five strategies that can be used to prevent trauma in adolescents.
5. Develop a chart that shows the differences between limb sprains and fractures and the patient care management needs of both.

APPENDIX A

Glossary

ACLS—advanced cardiac life support; emergency first aid that includes basic cardiac life support plus the use of drugs and adjunctive therapies, such as ventilation and defibrillation, to restore cardiac function

Amniotomy—artificial rupture of the fetal membranes

Antigen—substance that causes an antibody

Anxiety—vague, uneasy feeling caused by a nonspecific threat, real or imagined; the intensity of the feeling may range from mild to severe panic

Arrhythmia—abnormal cardiac rhythm

Asterixis—flapping tremor of hands with finger flexion

Atony—absence of muscle tone

Autoregulation—ability of vessels to alter their diameter to balance blood flow with metabolic demands

Balloon tamponade—catheter device with a balloon that, when inflated, exerts pressure on bleeding varices in the esophagus or stomach

BCLS—basic cardiac life support; emergency first aid focusing on identifying respiratory or cardiac arrest and providing cardiopulmonary resuscitation

Bigeminy—rhythm in which every other beat is a premature ventricular contraction

Brudzinski's sign—assessment technique used to determine the presence of meningitis; it is considered positive when forward flexion of the neck causes hip and knee flexion

Calibrate—to apply a known quantity of pressure to a transducer; the accuracy of the pressure measurement displayed can be evaluated with a built-in mechanism on the monitor or with a fluid-filled or mercury manometer

Calipers—two-legged instrument used to measure distance and determine rhythm on a cardiac monitoring strip

Capillary hydrostatic pressure—pressure of fluid against the blood vessel walls

Cardiac output—measurement of cardiac performance calculated by multiplying the heart rate times the stroke volume

Cardiomegaly—hypertrophy of the heart

Cardioversion—timed or synchronized depolarization of the myocardial cells by an externally applied electric charge

Catheter-related sepsis—systemic infection that can occur from the insertion and placement of an indwelling catheter

Colloidal osmotic pressure—also called oncotic pressure; the pressure exerted by proteins in a solution

Compensation—immediate effort by the respiratory system to retain or remove carbon dioxide to balance the effects of increased or decreased bicarbonate levels, which present as metabolic acidosis or alkalosis; also, effort by the renal system (requiring hours to days) to retain or excrete bicarbonate to balance the effects of increased or decreased carbon dioxide levels, which present as respiratory acidosis or alkalosis

Concussion—injury caused by traumatic jarring of body tissue; common brain injury

Contusion—injury caused by traumatic bruising of body tissue; brain, chest, or abdominal injury

CPAP-continuous positive airway pressure; positive pressure exerted on the airways throughout the respiratory cycle; used as an adjunct to weaning and to prevent alveolar collapse

CPR—cardiopulmonary resuscitation, which includes mouth-to-mouth breathing and closed cardiac compressions

Cross-contamination—spread of infective organisms from one site or person to another

Culdocentesis—use of an incision or needle puncture through the vaginal wall to remove intraperitoneal fluid

Defibrillation—untimed depolarization of the myocardial cells by an externally applied electric charge; used to terminate chaotic cardiac activity and reestablish a normal rhythm

Demand mode pacing—a method of pacing that senses the patient's heart rate and fires only if the patient's rate falls below a preset rate

Diabetes mellitus—condition produced by an alteration in glucose metabolism or use, causing the patient to be insulin-deficient

Diffusion—passive movement of particles or solutes from an area of higher concentration to one of lower concentration

DNR—do not resuscitate; written order not to initiate resuscitative measures based on the patient's and family's request or the patient's clinical condition

Durable power of attorney—the written designation by an individual for another individual to act on his or her behalf; does not end when the person loses decision-making capacity (under state law)

Dysarthria—difficulty in speaking caused by impairment of innervated speech organs

Electrolytes—active chemical particles, positively or negatively charged, that form varying combinations in body fluids; concentrations of electrolytes are commonly expressed in milliequivalents

Epicardial—refers to the visceral layer of the pericardium that covers the heart and great vessels

Epidural space—space surrounding the dura mater directly below the skull

Exophthalmos—condition characterized by protrusion of the eyeballs, caused by hyperthyroidism

Fear—feeling caused by a specific threat, real or imagined; the patient can identify the object of fear; the intensity of the feeling may range from mild to severe panic

Fibrinolysis—destruction of fibrin by enzymatic digestion of cells

FIO_2—(fraction of inspired oxygen); ventilator setting that refers to the fraction of inspired oxygen; actually a decimal but usually recorded as a percentage

Flail chest—injury to the chest from a fracture of multiple ribs, a fracture of the ribs or sternum, or a fracture of three or more ribs in two or more places, creating a detached segment

Foramen of Monro—passage between the lateral and third ventricles within the brain; used as an internal landmark for leveling the intracranial pressure monitor transducer

Gastric residual—amount of stomach contents that remains and is aspirated by a feeding syringe; the amount indicates the effectiveness of gastric absorption

Glasgow coma scale—assessment tool that evaluates the patient's level of consciousness according to three categories: eye opening, motor response, and verbal response

Guaiac test—test to determine the presence of blood; it uses a reagent solution that turns blue when blood is present

Harris-Benedict equation—mathematical formula for determining caloric needs that takes into account the patient's weight in kilograms, height in centimeters, age in years, activity, and injury

Hemoptysis—blood in sputum

Herniation of the brain—protrusion of part of the brain through an abnormal opening

Hormones—chemicals secreted by the endocrine glands that regulate metabolic functions

Informed consent—permission for treatment given by the patient after he or she has received sufficient information to make a decision about his or her health care

Isoelectric—showing no variation in electric potential (refers to the flat line between each waveform on the hard copy)

Jaundice—yellow skin color that occurs because of elevated serum bilirubin levels

Kernig's sign—assessment technique used to determine the presence of meningitis; it is considered positive when attempts to flex the hip of a recumbent person produce painful spasms of the hamstring muscle and resistance to further leg extension at the knee

Ketonemia—ketones in blood

Ketosis—accumulation of ketone bodies in body tissues and fluids caused by the breakdown of fatty acids

Laparoscopy—internal examination of the abdomen by inserting a small telescope through the anterior abdominal wall and filling the abdomen with carbon dioxide, allowing visualization of the abdominal organs

Lead—graphic illustration of the electrical potential difference between two points on the skin surface

Leopold's maneuver—four palpation maneuvers of the mother's abdomen to evaluate fetal position

LVEDP—pressure in the left ventricle at the end of diastole just before systolic contraction; it closely approximates the mean pulmonary arterial wedge pressure in the absence of mitral valve disease

Malpractice—act of omission or commission in which the nurse fails to conform to an identified standard of practice and causes the patient harm; it may include such acts as failing to observe or report changes in the patient's condition, failing to obtain informed consent, or administering the wrong drug to a patient

Melena—black, tarlike stool

Nephrotoxic—toxic or destructive to the kidneys

NIF—negative inspiratory force; measurement to demonstrate the muscle power needed to provide a tidal volume of 5 ml/kg; must be greater than -20 cm H_2O for spontaneous breathing to meet bodily needs

Oscilloscope—screen that displays the ECG tracing

Osmolality—concentration of a solution based on the number of particles in the solution

Osmosis—process of water movement across a semipermeable membrane in response to osmotic pressure; water moves from an area of lower solute concentration to one of higher concentration

PEEP—positive end-expiratory pressure; pressure exerted by mechanical ventilation at the end of expiration that keeps alveoli and small airways open to promote gas exchange

Phlebostatic axis—imaginary line, drawn where the fourth intercostal space intersects with the midaxillary line, that serves as the reference point for the right atrium

Pneumothorax—condition characterized by free air in the thoracic cavity, usually in the pleura, that has escaped from an opening in lung tissue; can result in tension pneumothorax with positive pressure ventilation and lead to mediastinal shift, which imposes on the unaffected lung and vascular structures

Polyphagia—excessive eating, a classic symptom of diabetes

Powerlessness—perceived lack of control over a situation that an individual believes that his or her actions cannot alter

Ptosis—abnormal drooping of the upper eyelid

Pulsus alternans—pulse characterized by a regular alternation of strong and weak beats

Resistant organism—organism that is insensitive to a prescribed antibiotic

Respiratory acidosis—acid-base imbalance occurring because of hypoventilation and retention of carbon dioxide

Respiratory alkalosis—acid-base imbalance occurring because of hyperventilation and excessive loss of carbon dioxide

Rhinorrhea—leakage of cerebrospinal fluid through the nose; commonly seen with a cranial fracture

Risk factors—characteristic findings associated with increased prevalence of a disease; modifiable risk factors for cardiovascular disease include cigarette smoking, hyperlipidemia, elevated blood pressure, elevated blood glucose levels, obesity, inactivity, and stress

R-on-T phenomenon—premature depolarization (R wave) that occurs during the relative refractory period of repolarization (T wave) of the preceding cycle; can trigger ventricular tachycardia or fibrillation

S_3 or S_4 heart sounds—abnormal heart sounds occurring during diastole that result from resistance to ventricular filling

SaO_2—percentage of saturation of hemoglobin in arterial blood; may be monitored noninvasively by pulse oximetry

Septicemia—systemic disease process caused by microorganisms and their toxic products in the blood

Sick sinus syndrome—a syndrome characterized by a combination of sinus block, sinus arrest, sinus bradycardia, and sinus tachycardia that interferes with cerebral perfusion, causing syncope and other cerebral dysfunctions

Starling's law—principle stating that the force of contraction depends on the length of the heart wall's muscle fibers. The more the muscles are stretched, the greater the force of contraction within physiologic limits

Surfactant—lipoprotein that decreases surface tension of the cell membrane and prevents alveolar collapse

Telemetry—means of continuous cardiac monitoring for an ambulatory patient, using a battery-powered generator that transmits the signal to a central stationary monitor screen

Territoriality—desire or need to possess and occupy a space and, if necessary, to defend it against intrusion from others

Tidal volume—amount of air breathed in or out with each breath

Transducer—device that converts the pressure transmitted by the fluid-filled tubing into an electrical signal represented by waveforms on an oscilloscope

Triage—method of decision making used by emergency nurses to determine which patients should be treated first and where treatment should take place

Unipolar lead—wire consisting of only one electrode

Volume pressure response—test for intracranial elastance and compliance performed by a doctor; sterile saline solution is injected into the intraventricular catheter or subarachnoid screw, and changes in pressure readings are recorded to assess altered compensation

Zero reference point—point at which air and fluid meet; physiologic pressures are relative to atmospheric pressure, so transducers must be balanced (zeroed) at atmospheric pressure

APPENDIX B

Answers to Study Questions

CHAPTER 1

1. Critical care and emergency nurses routinely make life-and-death decisions for which they are legally responsible, and they are at risk of exposure to communicable diseases, such as hepatitis, tuberculosis, and acquired immunodeficiency syndrome.
2. Certification in critical care nursing is available for adult, neonatal, and pediatric nursing.
3. The national emergency telephone number is 911; it provides access to EMS and other emergency services, such as police and fire departments.

CHAPTER 2

1. Normal ABG values are as follows: pH, 7.35 to 7.45; $PaCO_2$, 35 to 45 mm Hg; HCO_3^-, 22 to 26 mEq/liter; PaO_2, 80 to 100 mm Hg; SaO_2, 95% to 100%; base excess, -2.5 to +25.
2. The kidneys perform major regulatory functions, including retention and excretion of fluids and select electrolytes, regulation of pH and excretion of metabolic waste and toxic substances, and secretion of renin in response to decreased blood pressure or ECF volume.
3. Inadequate tissue perfusion activates several key compensatory mechanisms. Baroreceptors in the carotid and aortic arch stimulate the vasomotor center in the medulla. The sympathetic nervous system releases epinephrine and norepinephrine. Blood is shunted to vital organs and away from organs that tolerate ischemia. The respiratory rate increases to improve oxygenation. The renin-angiotensin-aldosterone system is activated — and the posterior pituitary gland secretes ADH — to increase water retention.
4. Gas exchange takes place in the alveoli.

CHAPTER 3

1. The patient typically experiences three stages in the cycle of health and illness: first, a transition from health to illness when the patient and family experience denial, disbelief, or shock; second, a developing awareness and acceptance that the patient needs help from others; third, a reorganizational period during which the patient gains renewed interest in life and makes plans for the future.
2. Many types of stressors can affect the patient's basic coping mechanisms. Biologic stressors include an injury or illness, its severity, and the patient's perception of its significance. Psychosocial

stressors include interpersonal conflicts with family members, legal or financial hardships, and growth and developmental conflicts. Environmental stressors in the ED or ICU include unfamiliarity with the surroundings, sensory overload or deprivation, and isolation or restricted visitation.
3. Self-regulating interventions that may produce a balanced response to illness include relaxation, imagery, and music therapy.

CHAPTER 4

1. Alternate feeding methods that provide nutritional support include tube or enteral feedings, PPN, TPN, and parenteral lipid emulsions.
2. Assess nasogastric tube placement by injecting air while listening over the stomach with a stethoscope or by aspirating gastric contents.
3. To minimize the risk of infection for a patient receiving TPN, do not use the line to give blood, administer medications, or measure central venous pressure and do not allow a TPN solution to hang for more than 24 hours. Use a filter to prevent infusion of gross particles. Keep the solution refrigerated until administration. Check the label on fluids to ensure the correct name and concentrations.

CHAPTER 5

1. The most common cause of septicemia in critically ill patients is the insertion of intravascular devices.
2. Culture and sensitivity studies identify the organism responsible for the infection and the appropriate antibiotics to use for treatment.
3. Thorough hand washing — using vigorous friction under running water with standard soap — is the primary means of preventing infection transmission.

CHAPTER 6

1. The sequence for CPR is A-B-C. Open Airway. Restore Breathing by using mouth-to-mouth resuscitation or a ventilatory assistance device. Restore Circulation by using closed chest compressions.
2. The American Heart Association identifies two types of emergency life support: BCLS, which includes emergency first aid and CPR, and ACLS, which includes BCLS plus the use of adjunctive therapies to support ventilation, I.V. access for fluid and drug administration, cardiac monitoring, defibrillation, arrhythmia control, and postresuscitation care.
3. Gasping or absent respirations and no carotid pulse indicate a need for CPR.
4. For any patient requiring BCLS or ACLS, the nurse should document the sequence of therapies and interventions, along with the patient's response.

CHAPTER 7

1. Hemodynamic complications of mechanical ventilation result from increased intrathoracic pressure that impedes venous return, thereby decreasing cardiac output and increasing pulmonary artery wedge pressure.
2. The most widely used mechanical ventilators are positive-pressure, volume-cycled ventilators. They exert positive pressure on the airways, delivering a predetermined volume of gas over a predetermined time.
3. SIMV is the most commonly used mode of ventilation. It delivers a preset, mandatory tidal volume synchronized to the patient's inspiratory effort.
4. The following diagnostic test findings indicate the need for mechanical ventilation: $PaCO_2$, 50; PaO_2, 50; pH, 7.35; tidal volume, 5 ml/kg; NIF, -20 cm H_2O; minute volume, 10 liters/minute.
5. The patient on a mechanical ventilator should be suctioned when assessment reveals fluid, mucus, or obstruction in the airways. Activation of the alarms for high-pressure limits also may indicate the need for suctioning.
6. The following test findings indicate the patient's readiness to be weaned from mechanical ventilation: $PaCO_2$, 45; PaO_2, 60; pH, 7.35 to 7.45; NIF, -20 cm H_2O; tidal volume, 15 ml/kg; FIO_2, 40%.

CHAPTER 8

1. The preferred insertion site for arterial pressure monitoring is the radial artery.
2. A normal arterial waveform consists of a rapid, sharp upstroke; a dicrotic notch; and a clear end-diastole.
3. CVP represents the filling pressure or preload of the right ventricle or right ventricular end-diastolic pressure.
4. The balloon of a PA catheter should be left to deflate passively to prevent balloon rupture.
5. Continuous mixed $S\bar{v}O_2$ measurements assess the balance between oxygen supply and tissue demand for oxygen; they reflect the body's ability to meet tissue oxygen needs.

CHAPTER 9

1. ICP is determined by the components within the cranial vault, including brain tissue volume, CSF, and blood volume.
2. The nurse should maintain the transducer at the foramen of Monro.
3. C waves indicate intracranial compression.
4. Epidural monitoring poses less danger of infection than do other methods, and it monitors ICP without opening the dura.

CHAPTER 10

1. Cardiac monitoring is indicated to monitor a critically ill patient; to observe symptomatic arrhythmias or cardiac pathology; and to evaluate drug, fluid, or electrolyte therapy.

2. Cardiac monitoring has some limitations: it measures only electrical activity and is not an indicator of cardiac mechanical function; it must be correlated with the patient's clinical status; and it is not a substitute for a 12-lead diagnostic ECG.
3. Lead II (in which the positive electrode is placed at the left midclavicular line, at or below the fifth intercostal space, and the negative electrode is placed on the right shoulder, below the clavicle) produces an upright waveform with clear P waves.
4. A modified chest lead, MCL_1 (in which the positive electrode is placed at the fourth intercostal space, on the right sternal border, and the negative electrode is placed on the left shoulder, below the clavicle) produces an inverted waveform and offers more diagnostic advantages for identifying ectopy and blocks.

CHAPTER 11

1. Arrhythmias are caused by a disturbance in automaticity, conductivity, or automaticity and conductivity.
2. The five steps of arrhythmia interpretation are as follows: determine the rate; determine the rhythm; analyze the P wave; measure the PR interval; and measure the QRS duration.
3. Arrhythmias are classified as sinus, atrial, supraventricular, junctional, ventricular, or atrioventricular.
4. Common causes of bradycardia include sleep, sedation, increased vagal tone, and drug therapy with beta blockers or sympatholytics.
5. Common causes of tachycardia include increased activity, stress, pain, caffeine, and hypotension.
6. Second-degree Mobitz type II and third-degree AV blocks require insertion of a permanent pacemaker.
7. Characteristics of a PVC include an absent or a retrograde P wave; a QRS complex duration wider than 0.12 second and bizarre looking; and a T-wave deflection in the opposite direction of the QRS complex and followed by a compensatory pause.
8. Ventricular tachycardia, ventricular fibrillation, and asystole are lethal or life-threatening arrhythmias.

CHAPTER 12

1. Three routes commonly used to insert a temporary pacemaker are the transvenous (placed in contact with the endocardium through a major vein by way of a percutaneous stick or cutdown), epicardial (attached to the epicardium during cardiac surgery with the wires brought out through the skin in the mediastinal area), and external (anterior and posterior conducting pads are placed on the skin).
2. If the patient with a temporary pacemaker experiences a cardiac arrest, make sure the pacemaker is on, turn up the heart rate to at least 60 beats/minute, and adjust

the pacing threshold high enough to capture the myocardium (pacing spikes should be visible on the ECG monitor, followed by a QRS complex). Assess for pulse to ensure that electrical stimulus has generated mechanical activity.

3. The ICD consists of a pulse generator and lead system. It corrects lethal ventricular arrhythmias by continuously analyzing the patient's cardiac rhythm. On recognition of ventricular fibrillation or tachycardia, the ICD delivers up to five internal electrical discharges to terminate the arrhythmia.
4. Using the QRS complex of the ECG as its trigger, the IABP balloon (when properly timed) has numerous benefits: Inflating the balloon displaces blood in the aorta up into the coronary arteries and the major vessels of the head and downward to the renal arteries, enhancing arterial perfusion (diastolic augmentation). Deflating the balloon immediately before systole reduces the amount of pressure that must be overcome to eject blood from the ventricle, thereby decreasing myocardial oxygen consumption (afterload reduction).
5. The nurse may observe the following signs and symptoms of IABP catheter migration: decreased left radial pulse, sudden decrease in urine output, flank pain, dizziness, or sudden change in level of consciousness.
6. Clinical signs of the effectiveness of a VAD include increased blood pressure, cardiac output, and urine output; improved mental alertness and hemodynamic parameters; warm, dry skin; and palpable peripheral pulses.

CHAPTER 13

1. Modifiable risk factors include cigarette smoking, hypertension, increased serum cholesterol levels, and diabetes. Contributing risk factors include obesity, physical inactivity, type A personality, and stress.
2. Coronary artery perfusion occurs during diastole.
3. Angina is commonly precipitated by physical exercise, stress, cold, heavy meals, or smoking; the pain usually subsides in 2 to 5 minutes with rest, nitroglycerin, or both. An MI may be asymptomatic or may produce substernal, crushing chest pain that sometimes radiates to the jaw, shoulders, back, and arms. The pain lasts longer than 30 minutes and is unrelieved by rest, position, or nitroglycerin.
4. Key tests used to diagnose an acute MI include serum enzyme studies and ECG readings. The CK-MB isoenzyme elevation is greater than institutional criterion, beginning 4 to 8 hours after infarction, peaking at 24 hours, and lasting for 72 hours after infarction. The LDH_1 level is greater than LDH_2 level, developing 12 to 24 hours after infarction, peaking at 36 to 72 hours, and returning to normal within 10 days after infarction.

ECG changes occur in leads over the area of infarction. ST-segment elevation indicates injury to myocardial tissue. ST-segment depression (in leads that view the opposite wall) and T-wave flattening and inversion indicate ischemia of the myocardial tissue. A Q wave (representing death of the tissue) is clinically significant if it is greater than one-third of the total QRS height or wider than 0.04 second.

5. Common assessment findings in left-sided heart failure are a moist cough with frothy sputum, dyspnea, crackles, S_3 or S_4 heart sounds, anxiety, diaphoresis, decreased blood pressure, tachycardia, arrhythmias, and pulsus alternans.
6. Medications commonly used to maintain hemodynamic stability in a patient with cardiomyopathy include vasodilators (to decrease preload and afterload, thereby improving CO), diuretics (to reduce preload and pulmonary congestion), inotropic agents (to increase contractility), calcium channel blockers (to decrease cardiac workload through vasodilation), beta blockers (for hypertrophic cardiomyopathy to reduce outflow obstruction during exercise), and anticoagulants (to prevent clot formation associated with atrial fibrillation).
7. Medical and surgical interventions used to treat cardiac tamponade include pericardiocentesis or pericardiostomy to drain pericardial space of excess fluid; I.V. volume therapy with fluids and volume expanders to increase diastolic filling pressure and improve CO; oxygen at a flow rate based on the patient's clinical condition to correct hypoxia; administration of inotropic agents to increase contractility; and resuscitative measures, if necessary.
8. Nitroprusside is the drug of choice for treating hypertensive crisis.

CHAPTER 14

1. The major management goal for a patient with a respiratory disorder is to maintain a patent airway.
2. The normal stimulus for respiration is an increase in the partial pressure of carbon dioxide in arterial blood.
3. Sputum characteristics that the nurse should observe for and document include color, viscosity, quantity, and odor.
4. The primary auscultatory finding in a patient with status asthmaticus is prolonged expiratory wheezing; absence of wheezing indicates insufficient airflow or respiratory collapse.
5. Heparin (given initially as a bolus, followed by a continuous infusion) is the drug of choice for pulmonary embolus caused by a clot.
6. The auscultatory findings characteristic of emphysema include decreased lung sounds and prolonged expiration.

7. Patients with COPD are more difficult to wean from mechanical ventilation because they retain higher levels of carbon dioxide, which depresses the respiratory drive.
8. Reported cases of tuberculosis have increased since 1981, primarily because of immunosuppression and an increase in the elderly population.

CHAPTER 15

1. The three key functions of the renal system are regulation of acid, water, and electrolyte excretion.
2. Causes of metabolic acidosis include diabetic ketoacidosis, starvation, renal failure, poisoning, diarrhea, lactic acidosis, intestinal fistulas, and administration of large amounts of normal saline solution or ammonium chloride.
3. The ABG findings that differentiate uncompensated metabolic acidosis from compensated metabolic acidosis are a decreased $Pa{CO_2}$ level and a pH that approximates normal.
4. ECG changes are the most reliable indicator of potassium imbalance.
5. ECG changes associated with hypokalemia include flat T waves and ST-segment depression. ECG changes associated with hyperkalemia include widening QRS complex; tall, tented T waves; and asystole. With hypercalcemia, ECG changes include a shortened QT interval and arrhythmias. ECG changes associated with hypocalcemia include a prolonged QT interval.
6. Common causes of fluid volume deficit are insufficient intake of water and electrolytes, excessive fluid loss through secretions or excretions, and third-space shifting.
7. The most common cause of acute renal failure is acute tubular necrosis.

CHAPTER 16

1. Hormones regulate the transport of chemicals, chemical reactions, and growth functions in the body.
2. Assessment findings observed in DKA include dry, flushed skin; fruity breath odor; rapid and deep respirations; polydipsia; polyphagia; and polyuria.
3. Initial management of DKA includes administration of regular insulin (given first as a bolus, followed by a continuous infusion to decrease serum glucose levels); infusion of normal saline solution; I.V. fluids until the serum glucose level is 200 to 300 mg/dl; and use of solutions containing glucose.
4. Ketonemia does not occur in HHNS because insulin is present in amounts adequate to prevent ketosis (but not to prevent hyperglycemia).
5. The initial goal for management of hypoglycemia is to elevate the serum glucose level promptly, either by administering 50% glucose I.V. if the patient is unconscious or by feeding fast-acting carbohydrates (such as fruit

juices, honey, sugar, and corn syrup) if the patient is conscious.
6. The cause of SIADH is uncontrolled production or excessive secretion of ADH.
7. The kidneys attempt to compensate for excessive water retention caused by SIADH by filtering more sodium into the concentrated urine, which results in severe hyponatremia.
8. DI is caused by inadequate secretion of ADH, most commonly as the result of head injury or trauma to the posterior pituitary.
9. Aspirin should not be given for fever control in thyrotoxicosis because it replaces T_3 from carrier proteins and increases the free T_3 levels.

CHAPTER 17

1. The two compensatory mechanisms that protect the brain under adverse conditions are collateral circulation, which allows for alternate blood flow if normal blood flow is occluded; and autoregulation, which maintains constant blood flow through vasodilation or constriction stimulated by serum carbon dioxide, oxygen concentration, and arterial blood pressure.
2. Common assessment findings in a patient with a left CVA include right hemiparesis or hemiplegia; right homonymous hemianopia; memory deficits in language; expressive or receptive aphasia; slow, cautious behavior; and acute intellectual impairment. Common assessment findings in a patient with a right CVA include left hemiparesis or hemiplegia; left homonymous hemianopia; memory deficits in performance; impulsive behavior; lack of motivation; and spacial-perceptual deficits.
3. The key diagnostic test for meningitis is a lumbar puncture, which identifies the type of causative agent by abnormality of glucose, protein, and WBC count.
4. The brain compensates for increases in ICP by regulating the intracranial volume, displacing CSF into the spinal canal, and increasing or decreasing CSF production.

CHAPTER 18

1. The distal section of the esophagus is the most common site of esophageal varices.
2. Vasopressin, a drug of choice for treating esophageal varices, constricts mesenteric, splenic, and hepatic arterioles, resulting in decreased blood flow to the portal system.
3. Tension or traction is placed on the balloon tamponade device when the esophageal balloon is deflated for two reasons: to maintain its position in the esophagus and to prevent movement upward to the oropharynx, where it could occlude the airway.
4. The causes of lower GI hemorrhage include ruptured diverticula and ischemic bowel polyps, tumors, and eroding aortic aneurysm.

5. Trypsinogen, a pancreatic enzyme, initiates autodigestion of the pancreas, which results in pancreatitis.
6. Meperidine hydrochloride, the narcotic of choice for pain management in pancreatitis, causes fewer spasms of pancreatic and biliary ducts than morphine.

CHAPTER 19

1. Most ectopic pregnancies occur in the fallopian tubes, more commonly in the right than in the left.
2. Placenta previa presents with the following assessment findings: painless uterine bleeding, especially in the third trimester; normal uterine tone; Leopold's maneuver with the fetus in breech, oblique, or transverse position; and port wine amniotic fluid.
3. Premature separation of the placenta from the uterine wall begins when the small arteries in the uterine wall degenerate, rupture, and hemorrhage, causing a severe decrease in blood flow to the placenta. The uterus cannot contract and compress the torn vessels effectively, and hemorrhage continues.
4. PIH is a leading cause of maternal mortality.
5. $MgSO_4$ is the drug of choice as an anticonvulsant. Before administering $MgSO_4$, check the patient's reflexes (knee, ankle, biceps), urine output, and respirations. Do not administer the drug if reflexes are absent, urine output is less than 100 ml in the previous 4 hours, or respirations are fewer than 12 per minute to prevent potentially life-threatening adverse reactions. Have the antidote, calcium gluconate, available.

CHAPTER 20

1. In a patient with early septic shock, assessment findings include tachycardia; systolic blood pressure less than 90 mm Hg (or 30 mm Hg less than baseline); CO less than 4 liters/minute; SVR less than 1,200 dynes/sec/cm^{-5}; tachypnea; $Paco_2$ greater than 45 mm Hg; decreasing body temperature; urine output less than 30 ml/hour; and changes in LOC.
2. The physiologic processes that predispose a patient to hemorrhage in DIC are coagulation, anticoagulation, and fibrinolysis.
3. The extrinsic and the intrinsic coagulation pathways are activated in DIC.
4. HIV is responsible for causing AIDS.
5. A retrovirus, HIV incorporates itself into normal cell ribonucleic acid, destroying normal T4 helper cells and cells with a CD4 molecule (monocytes).
6. The Rule of Nines provides a quick method of estimating the extent of an adult patient's burns, expressed as a percentage of body surface area. To use this method, calculate the corresponding percentage for each burned body section: the head and neck (9%), upper extremities (18%), the anterior (18%) and posterior torso (36%), each

lower extremity (18%), and the perineum (1%).

CHAPTER 21

1. An acceleration head injury occurs when a moving object strikes the head; a deceleration head injury occurs when the head strikes a stationary object.
2. Decerebrate posturing or abnormal extension can be seen in a patient with a head injury involving the brain stem.
3. Assessment findings in head injuries commonly include altered LOC, nausea, vomiting, and headache.
4. Elevating the head of the bed facilitates cerebral venous return and helps control ICP.
5. Nonnarcotic analgesics are used for pain management in chest and abdominal trauma to avoid respiratory depression and altered sensorium.
6. The immediate nursing action for wound evisceration is to cover the wound with a sterile, wet saline dressing but not to attempt to replace the eviscerated tissue.
7. The immediate patient management goal for limb trauma is to immobilize the affected area and prevent further injury.
8. Diagnostic test findings that can be used as legal evidence in a rape case include aspirated or scraped specimens from involved orifices and the patient's clothing; pubic hair scrapings; and fingernail scrapings.

APPENDIX C

Identifying and Treating Arrhythmias

The following chart highlights the characteristics, causes and underlying mechanisms, and treatments of arrhythmias commonly seen by critical care nurses.

ARRHYTHMIA/ CHARACTERISTICS	CAUSES/UNDERLYING MECHANISMS	TREATMENT
Sinus bradycardia		
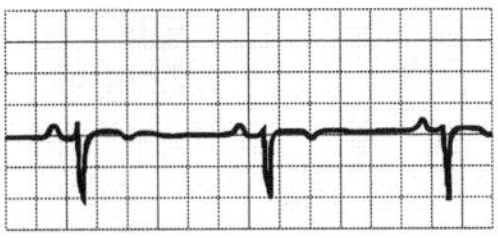 • Regular • P waves normal • AV rates < 60/minute • PR interval normal • QRS complex normal	• Impulse originates in sinus node more slowly than usual • Vagal stimulation, beta blockers, calcium channel blockers, ischemia, myocardial infarction (MI)	• Treat only if symptomatic. • Atropine increases sinus rate, resulting in relief of symptoms. • Consider pacemaker if condition persists.
Sinus tachycardia		
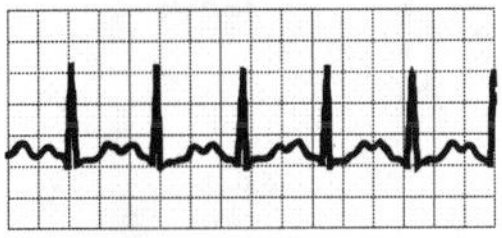 • Regular • P waves normal • AV rates > 100/minute • PR interval normal • QRS complex normal	• Impulse originates in sinus node more quickly than usual • Exercise, stress, pain, fever, strong emotion, hypovolemia, MI	• Treat underlying cause.
Premature atrial complex (PAC)		
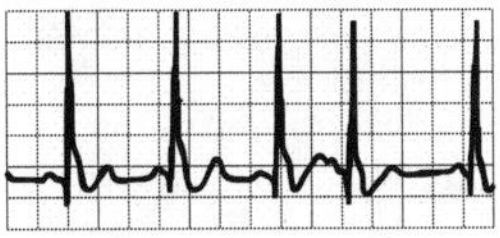 • Irregular • P waves present; premature P waves may differ in shape and may be hidden in preceding T wave • AV rates depend on underlying rhythm • PR interval may be normal, short, or prolonged • QRS complex normal	• Ectopic site within atrium initiates beat before next sinus beat • May be normal if infrequent; frequent PACs due to atrial strain (in congestive heart failure [CHF]), ischemia, or mechanical irritation (cannulation for heart-lung bypass)	• Consider treating if > 6/minute, as this may indicate irritability that may lead to atrial fibrillation or atrial flutter. • Administer type 1A antiarrhythmics (quinidine, procainamide).

ARRHYTHMIA/ CHARACTERISTICS	CAUSES/UNDERLYING MECHANISMS	TREATMENT
Atrial fibrillation (A-fib)		
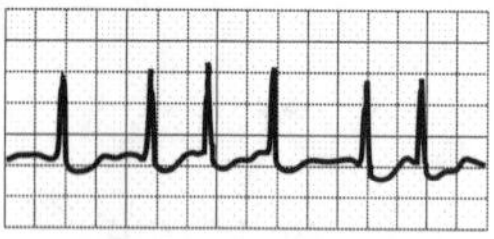 • Irregular • No P waves; atrial activity is coarse or fine fibrillatory waves • Atrial rate 375 to 600/minute; ventricular rate 30 to > 200/minute • No PR interval • QRS complex usually normal	• Multiple foci in atria simultaneously initiate impulses with only a small area of tissue responding to each; atria do not contract in a coordinated fashion, but rather quiver • Mechanical irritation, atrial strain (from CHF or chronic obstructive pulmonary disease)	• Quinidine, procainamide, or amiodarone may suppress the ectopic foci. • Digoxin increases chance of remaining in sinus rhythm in the event of conversion. • I.V. verapamil or diltiazem hydrochloride will control a fast ventricular rate. • Pacing cardioversion or synchronized electrical cardioversion may be needed. • Some patients with enlarged atria will remain in A-fib.
Atrial flutter (A-flutter)		
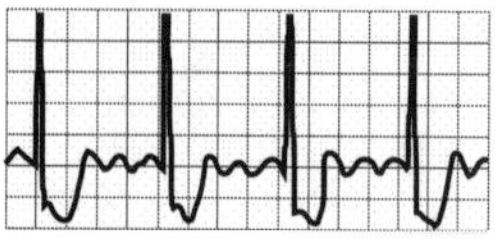 • Regular or irregular • No P waves; atrial activity is regular flutter waves ("sawtooth" baseline) • Atrial rate 275 to 350/minute; ventricular rate depends on ratio of conduction • No PR interval • QRS complex may be distorted by flutter waves	• Reentry focus within the atria • Mechanical irritation, atrial strain	• Vagal maneuvers may slow ventricular rate so flutter waves are visible. • I.V. verapamil or diltiazem will control fast ventricular rate. • Quinidine, procainamide, and digoxin may alter reentry pathway. • Synchronized electrical cardioversion needed.
Supraventricular tachycardia (SVT)		
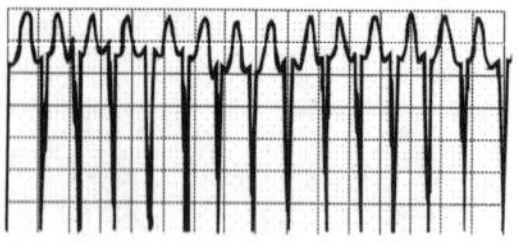 • Regular • P waves present but may be hidden • AV rates > 100/minute • PR interval constant; may be normal, short, or long • QRS complex usually normal	• May be sinus tachycardia, paroxysmal atrial tachycardia, rapid A-flutter, or junctional tachycardia; "SVT" is used generically until further evidence allows more accurate rhythm identification	• Try vagal maneuvers to slow or convert rhythm. • I.V. adenosine or procainamide may convert rhythm. • Synchronized electrical cardioversion may be needed.

ARRHYTHMIA/ CHARACTERISTICS	CAUSES/UNDERLYING MECHANISMS	TREATMENT
Premature ventricular complex (PVC)		
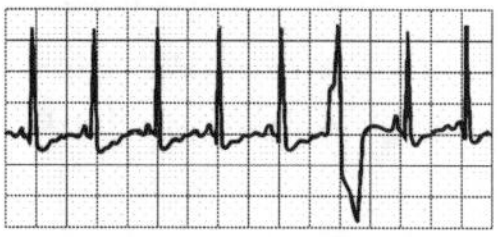 • Irregular • Usually no P wave before PVC • Rates depend on underlying rhythm • PR interval not measured for PVC • QRS complex wide, generally > 0.16 second	• Ectopic focus in ventricle fires before next sinus beat • Electrolyte imbalance (especially hypokalemia), ischemia, MI, catecholamines, cardiomyopathy, abnormal electrical function at border of MI scar	• Consider treating if > 6/minute, increasing frequency, occurring in couplets, triplets, or bigeminy. • Treat with antiarrhythmic drugs. • Treat underlying cause.
Ventricular tachycardia (V-tach)		
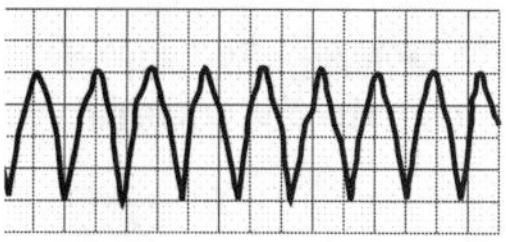 • Regular • P waves present but rarely seen; if seen, are not associated with QRS complex • Ventricular rate > 100/minute • No PR interval • QRS complex wide, > 0.10 second	• Reentry mechanism in ventricles • Ischemia, cardiomyopathy, MI, electrolyte imbalance, abnormal function in tissue bordering MI scar or ventricular aneurysm • Long QT interval (may be induced by type 1A antiarrhythmics)	• Assess patient. • If stable, begin I.V. lidocaine. • If unstable (chest pain, severe dyspnea, hypotension), begin sedation and synchronized cardioversion. • If pulseless, defibrillate and begin CPR.
Ventricular fibrillation (V-fib)		
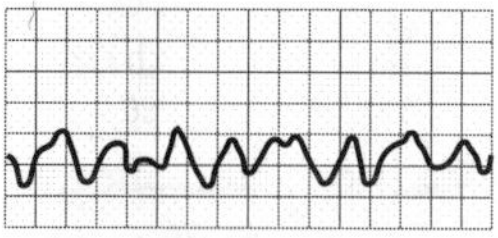 • Irregular • No P waves • No rate • No PR interval • No QRS complex, chaotic electrical activity	• Multiple foci in ventricles initiating beats, no coordinated contraction so no cardiac output • Fibrillatory waves may be coarse or fine; coarse waves are more likely to be converted • MI, severe hypoxia, severe acidosis	• Defibrillate. • Begin CPR. • I.V. epinephrine will increase amplitude of waves and increase chance of successful defibrillation.
Asystole		
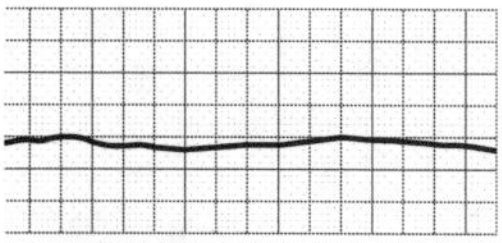 • No rhythm • No P waves • No AV rate • No PR interval • No QRS complex • "Flat line"	• Failure of all pacemakers • MI, severe hypoxia, severe acidosis	• Begin CPR. • I.V. atropine or epinephrine may restore some electrical activity. • Temporary pacemaker may be needed.

Selected References

Ahrens, T. *Critical Care Certification Preparation and Review,* 3rd ed. Norwalk, Conn.: Appleton & Lange, 1993.

Alspach, J., and Williams, S. *Core Curriculum for Critical Care Nursing,* 4th ed. Philadelphia: W.B. Saunders Co., 1991.

American Association of Critical Care Nurses. *Standards for Nursing Care of the Critically Ill,* edited by Sarah J. Sanford and Joanne M. Disch. Norwalk, Conn.: Appleton & Lange, 1989.

EmergiCare Cards. Springhouse, Pa.: Springhouse Corp., 1996.

Garner, Julia S. "Guideline for Isolation Precautions in Hospitals," *Infection Control and Hospital Epidemiology* 17(1), January 1996.

Hudak, C.M., *Critical Care Nursing: A Holistic Approach,* 5th ed. Philadelphia: J.B. Lippincott Co., 1994.

Larsen, Elaine L. "APIC Guidelines for Handwashing and Hand Antisepsis in Health Care Settings," *American Journal of Infection Control* 23(4), August 1995.

Kinney, M., et al. *AACN Clinical Reference for Critical Care Nursing.* New York: McGraw-Hill Book Co., 1993.

Shannon, M.T., and Wilson, B.A., eds. *Govoni and Hayes: Drugs and Nursing Implications,* 8th ed. Norwalk, Conn.: Appleton & Lange, 1995.

Sheehy, S.B., and Barber, J. *Emergency Nursing: Principles and Practice,* 2nd ed. St. Louis: Mosby, Inc., 1992.

Swearingen, P.L., et al. *Manual of Critical Care: Applying Nursing Diagnosis to Adult Critical Illness,* 3rd ed. St. Louis: Mosby, Inc., 1995.

Thelan, L.A., et al. *Textbook of Critical Care Nursing: Diagnosis and Management,* 2nd ed. St. Louis: Mosby, Inc., 1993.

Thomas, Judy Selfridge, and Shea, Sheila Sanning. *Emergency Nursing Standards of Care and Quality Improvement.* Philadelphia: W.B. Saunders Co., 1994.

Index

i refers to an illustration; t refers to a table

i refers to an illustration; t refers to a table

i refers to an illustration; t refers to a table

i refers to an illustration; t refers to a table

About the StudySmart Disk

StudySmart Disk lets you:

- review subject areas of your choice and learn the rationales for the correct answers
- take tests of varying lengths on subjects of your choice
- print the results of your tests to gauge your progress over time.

Recommended system requirements
486 IBM-compatible personal computer (386 minimum)
Windows 3.1 or greater (Windows 95 compatible)
High-density 3½″ floppy drive
8 MB RAM (4 MB minimum)
S-VGA monitor (VGA minimum)
2 MB of available space on hard drive

Installing and running the program

- Start Windows.
- In Program Manager, choose Run from File menu.
- Insert disk, type a:\setup.exe (where a: is the letter of your floppy drive), and click on OK.

For Windows 95 Installation

- Start Windows.
- Select Start button and then Run.
- Insert disk, type a:\setup.exe (where a: is the letter of your floppy drive), and click on OK.

For technical support, call 215-628-7744 Monday through Friday, 9 a.m. to 6 p.m. Eastern Standard Time.

The clinical information and tools in the *StudySmart Disk* are based on research and consultation with nursing, medical, and legal authorities. To the best of our knowledge, this program reflects currently accepted practice; nevertheless, it can't be considered absolute or universal. For individual application, all recommendations must be considered in light of the patient's clinical condition and, before administration of new or infrequently used drugs, in light of the latest package-insert information. The authors and publisher disclaim responsibility for any adverse effects resulting directly or indirectly from the suggested procedures, from any undetected errors, or from the reader's misunderstanding of the program.

Springhouse Corporation warrants to the user that the program media on which the software is recorded shall be free from defects in materials and workmanship for a period of ninety (90) days from the date of the user's purchase. Springhouse Corporation's liability shall be limited to correction or replacement of defective media.

This book cannot be returned for credit or refund if the vinyl disk holder has been opened, broken, or otherwise tampered with.